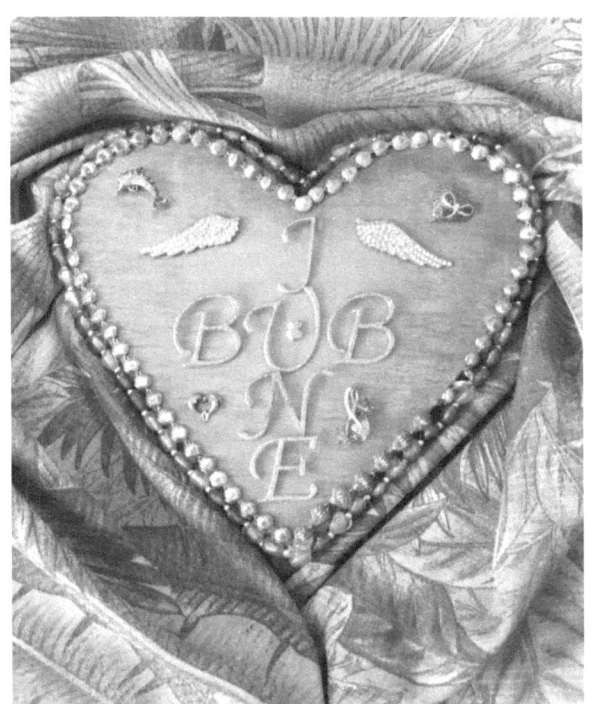

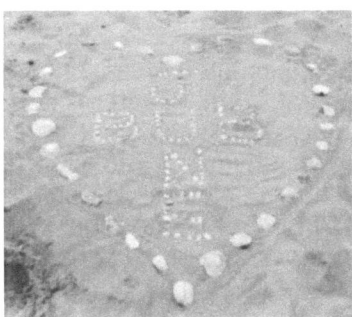

Newer version above of old standard beach visits shell sculpture tribute of Bub's love for June.

AMBUSH

PREFACE

I began this semi autobiography of my life following an illness caused by my exposure to agent orange as a result of my being drafted into the Vietnam war in 1969. Feeling that small portion of my life in chronological time was very large by comparison in personal development, and doubtless, the most difficult part of my life to that point, I hoped it would steel me from future difficult times. My VA counselor and I felt this would be a therapeutical exercise and I decided to get started several years ago, after much of her friendly persuasion.

I found over the years that I was to be further tested in ways I did not think possible, the most devastating when my wife June, of 42 years and best friend for 46, died from complications of cancer. Suddenly, I had been splashed into a deep black pool of depression, much more harsh than what I thought I endured when I left her behind after being married only seven months prior to boarding a plane destined for Vietnam almost 43 years earlier.

I roughed my writings out in three distinct sections when I began: The Beginning, Vietnam and Hallucinations, jumping from one to the other, not thinking of it as one story, but three while trying to cull my life into all three sections to encapsulate the entirety. As a result, the formal sequential and chronological norm for books is not practical for my brand of story telling, as my friends know, I tend to digress often and bounce around as new subjects are breached or pop into my head, thus my unusual writing style.

I apologize if this style of writing is hard for people to follow, but I did not want to just assign arbitrary chapters to the writing, but depict it as it came from my thoughts and memories of my experiences as well as my dreams and hallucinations included further on.

I decided to begin at the point of discovering my illness at age sixty-one and build three distinct books within one title, joined with and enclosed in the roving personal story of my life, prevalent throughout the book, but only hinted at in the hallucinations portion.

The first two books also envelop some of the personal history of my time in Vietnam and my own, non political views from those experiences and future knowledge gained from books and documentaries. I stress non political, because I am not a political person, nor have I ever been and have always based my opinions and reactions to events on what I decide is true or not true, right or wrong, good or bad, determined largely on my common sense. Those tools I use as my own personal judge, with the final test of looking at the person in the mirror and being able to evaluate my actions and feelings and finally, to live with myself.

In searching my mind for a title to both incorporate the sections and add value to the three dramatic experiences added to my Vietnam experience, I settled on the "war terminology", AMBUSH. Self explanatory in a section of Book II: Vietnam, I wanted to provide the harsh feelings of the other three incidences and how substantially they have impacted my life by following suit and naming those events as ambushes (surprise attacks) upon myself also.

Book I: The Beginning, contains my struggle with illnesses and starts thirty seven years after returning from Vietnam with my diagnosis and is depicted in Section I, Ambush by Agent Orange and contains a good bit of the biography and the beginning of the book sequentially. Section II, Ambush by Cancer includes June's diagnosis of breast cancer and her avalanche of problems and disease during her final two years. While the beginning of the writing, it contains the second and third chronological traumatic events in the story of my actual life, in relation to my ambushes.

Book II: Vietnam is obvious and falls second in book sequence, but first in my life ambush sequence and the primary basis of the title. It details that initial separation period of our lives, but expands the biography by relating to some of the events experienced while in country as well as much of the developmental views I lived with and enhanced over the rest of my life, with current views of some of life's issues which I'm sure will provoke strong feelings both ways. I wanted to stay away from the typical personal individual war stories of which I am so well read, and enjoy so much, as well as make the events in country less about me and more about my feelings and thoughts, but do include some of the most pivotal personal times in Section III, Ambush by NVA.

Book III: Hallucinations, and Section IV, Ambush by Hallucinations focuses on a very minute portion of the actual events surrounding three hospitalizations incurred around the first Christmas following June's passing and roughly two year increments centering on the anniversaries of her passing. I indicate small portion, because I have such total recall of most of those times, involving more than forty personas involved in my life's memories and my mind's concoctions via those events and associated conversations, that I could fill volumes. My intent was to instill a vivid picture of what I was experiencing in my head and in actuality and sometimes blurring together, during those times at home, in the hospital and back home again, without being totally inclusive and too personal, and leaving out some of the more sadistic and embarrassing examples.

This final period of the book and my life is these most recent six years of my life and hopefully the last to include "ambushes". These three periods of time and the final home recuperation period depict the accelerating and sequential course of events that evolved into my freakishly close suicide attempt resulting in my self admittance into a VA mental health facility, following my driving myself to the local ER and being admitted into ICU for four days, and subsequent transfer.

The four subtitled Ambush sections incorporated in the three books are my depiction, of the most dramatic and life changing events which happened to June and I during my life and 75% of hers. They have had much to do with how I got to where I am today and are shaped by meeting June at age 18 and that first Ambush by NVA at 23 years of age.

Most of these stories have not been shared with but a few people in my life in their entirety, and I have a mild hope that my personal experiences may help others in need, especially veterans and their families to possibly assist them toward a better life for themselves. Not just veterans with problems, people of specific age, or socioeconomic groups or any other distinction, but anyone in need of support of any kind.

I have definitely found that after sixty plus years of doubting that anyone other than myself, my wife or we as a team could help me with interpersonal challenges, that people are indeed available, willing to help pull you out of the fog, if you are game.

I eliminated some names and unit ID's in order for some anonymity, as well as workplaces, but I hope it still gives the air of reality and actual life experiences. I know that period of my life had profound and lasting effects on me and know that there are many, many similar stories out there and ready to be told. Take the leap and give it a shot, I'm sure you will feel better after sharing, I do.

Mentioned later in the writing is the fact that while growing up, my brother called me Bubba as he couldn't pronounce brother at a young age. I was called Bub or Bubba my entire life until my college days (before Bubba was popular) when I became James, Jim or Hackney, followed by the service and Sergeant, Hack, Hackney, or Delaware, to my work career, Mr., Jim or Bub, from old friends, and finally by Kyle and the six that followed, Bubby.

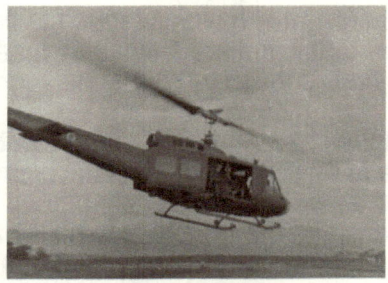

3rd Brigade, 101st Airborne Division
Command & Control Chopper
Huey UH 1

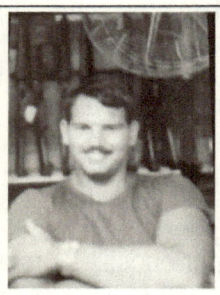
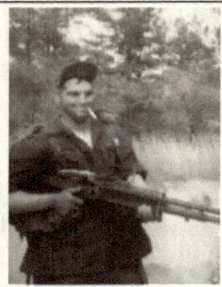

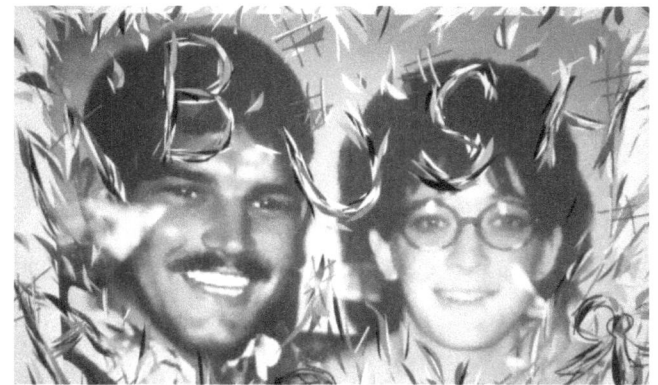

Bub & June, R & R Hawaii, April 1971

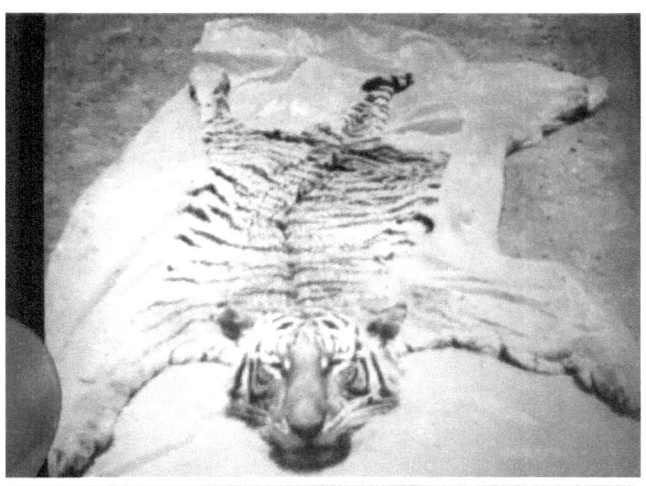

Tiger killed by mechanical ambush concussion only, no blood visible, by 101st in the A Shau Valley, Thua Thien Province, ICORP, SVN

DEDICATIONS

First, I would like to dedicate this undertaking to my late wife June, who I love and miss beyond belief and always will. She was beautiful and the love of my life from the time she was sweet sixteen and still was at age 62, and I think of the time we spent together constantly, while wishing that I could have done some things differently and better. She has always been my inspiration and kept me pushing to help her make the best life possible for us, our two children and seven grandchildren, and hopefully I have expressed as much in these writings, as it was always my personal goal to do everything I could to take care of her and keep her surprised, happy and cared for.

Secondly, I would like to thank Shannon and Chris, our children for their support to both of us during our hard times of need and my obnoxious behavior at times. I couldn't have gotten here without their support and love as well as their children, in order of their arrival into our family, Kyle, Kam, Isela, Kenzie, Buddy, Max and last but certainly not least, tiny Adriana. They are always there when I need to smile and loosen up my old joints and play games or watch movies and wrestle. June never got to see Max and Adriana, knew Buddy and Kenzie just as babies, but would have been tickled pink now with all of them, as she was with the first three. My, how she loved her grand babies, and her beautiful and handsome growing grands.

Next, thank you to the rest of my family and June's for helping me my entire life but especially during these past six lonely years. Also in this group, I would like to mention all of my lifelong friends as far back as grade school, and through my entire working career, including our children's friends. Many of them have been there with me through some good and bad times and have always supported me in the most kind and direct manner. I know they have been and always will be there in time of need as they have proven in the past. I have several spiritual connections there as well, and you know who you are along with June.

I can't dedicate this experience of remembering the past, without fondly recalling all of the people I served with in the Army, especially in Vietnam. To them and all who served and serve in the future as well as their families, I wish them the best luck available and encourage all veterans to be checked out for Agent Orange attributable diseases, of which I included a list and PTSD. The damage can be there for many years without notice or any indication, so protect yourself and your family. There are not enough words for the KIA, WIA and MIA's that suffered from our conflict, recent conflicts and will in future tragedies. They and their families can never be compensated adequately.

Finally, I want to personally thank all of my VA doctors, nurses and technicians that have watched over me for the past ten years and made my life more bearable and functional.

A very special thank you along with my full appreciation goes to my friend and counselor, as well as spiritual connection, Debra who was the driving force in getting me off my duff to begin and especially complete this project along with others as well. What drive, determination and commitment that woman has, and her dedication to her work and especially her charges, is unmatched in my experience. I owe much more to her than the appreciation for this book. She has been indispensable to me from the beginning, when my doctors and friends suggested I get help to deal with the loss of my lovely wife of forty-two years, June. I was a true skeptic, but now I suggest to friends in similar circumstances to search for help as competent as Debra. I wish them the best of luck with what they have facing them, and encourage them and especially veterans to reach out and obtain the assistance you so deserve.

TABLE OF CONTENTS

PREFACE	**1**
DEDICATIONS	**9**
TABLE OF CONTENTS	**12**
BOOK I: THE BEGINNING	**14**
SECTION I: AMB. BY A. ORANGE	20
SECTION II: AMB. BY CANCER	29
BOOK II: VIETNAM	**93**
SECTION III: AMBUSH BY NVA	162
BOOK III: HALLUCINATIONS	**186**
FIRST HOSPITAL ADMISSION	186
SECOND HOSPITAL ADMISSION	190
THIRD HOSPITAL ADMISSION	199
HOME RECUPERATION	213
GLOSSARY/BIBLIOGRAPHY:	**225**

Vietnam War Statistics   **225**

Vietnam Military Slang Glossary **227**

A. Orange Associated Diseases   **228**

The Viet Vet - Facts VS Fiction   **231**

Lam Som 719   **236**

The My Lai Massacre   **237**

Accelerationism   **238**

Doxorubicin Chemo Drug   **239**

AMBUSH
(My Life's Surprise Attacks)

BOOK I: THE BEGINNING

During and shortly after my tour in Vietnam (1970-1971) I realized that it would probably be the most difficult thing I would ever have to endure in my life. I had just finished four unremarkable years of college life and received my draft notice with two weeks of classes remaining. The one remarkable event during those four years was meeting and becoming engaged with my future wife June. I knew she was the one for me and I began working to make sure she felt the same way, or at least that she liked me. Having to begin transitioning to the Army way of life so soon and with knowing what was likely ahead, put a lot of pressure on us to try and do the right thing for both of us as we progressed with our relationship and plans.

Experiencing what was to be our future and legacy is reflected in these writings and is the basis of the rest of my life, and June's as well because we did decide to get married before I left for Vietnam, as there was little doubt of my travel plans, having been drafted. I will relive those nearly two years of separation from June, my new love and then my new wife, time and time again over the course of my life. All of the good and the not so good times were the foundation of our relationship and is what still carries me through to this day, now alone, without the girl, turned woman, mother and grandmother during forty-five wonderful years together, over in a flash, with some very rough times along the way.

Because of that, I have always convinced myself that there wasn't anything that could upset me in the future to the extent of my loneliness for her and the tough life experiences while in Vietnam. I had always been an optimistic person, but that only intensified the feeling of things not seeming so bad because of what I felt that I had been through. As the years wore on and I met our life's challenges, those feelings just became more relevant.

June and I opted to restart my career five times, a few, taking steps backward, to begin anew. One of those times the backward step was a huge financial change for the worse, others not quite so severe, and a few were positive, but we persisted while growing our family and managed together, to surpass each previous threshold. June's career was solid through the ten years of our courtship, the births of our daughter Shannon and son Chris, curtailed by a family move to the northern New Jersey mountains where she finally was able to start her stay at home Mom career, but obviously not with less work. Her career resumed following our return to Delaware three years later, as I began yet another career change which also required new areas of employment for her, but continuing in the medical clerical field as she began, transitioning into retail sales as time moved on, and finalized watching our first granddaughter, Isela, after she was born, until I became ill and taking care of me.

I am a very optimistic person and admit that I try to push my optimism toward those more cautious or pessimistic people, which I shouldn't do because they are where they are because of their own life experiences. I feel that it is better for the psyche to see the glass more full than empty because there is plenty of gloom and doom in the world without trying to find more. June and I continually discussed and often disagreed on that concept our entire life together, which escalated into arguments on occasion, as she often worried about what might possibly go wrong next. Too much of that in my opinion gives a person nothing positive to look forward to, only misery, and I don't know how anyone can deal with that on a steady basis, I know I can't, and do not try to fool myself or others, sometimes to a fault, and possibly causing ill feelings.

As hardships arise in my life, because of my mind set following my time in the service, I always try to convince myself that it will not be as bad as things I have already endured in my life, because I have already made it through worse times. That philosophy, and my well known stubbornness, and patience has helped carry me through all of them, but not without the support of family and friends, which I have been blessed with my entire life, June at the top of that list.

I also have quite a few Veteran friends that share that and other common philosophies and beliefs.
It is not lost on us, that the lessons learned when young, impressionable and possibly fearful of losing your life, or worse for me in particular, becoming a severe casualty, are lasting and useful throughout your life, and become a natural part of your personality. For better or worse, they are built into me and I believe help me overcome more than I think is sometimes possible for me. Other customs, habits and philosophies may not be so useful and respected, but we do have to take the good with the bad, don't we?

In short, like many veterans, and certainly June and I as well, our lives were thrust into a fast mode of learning life's secrets. We made life developing decisions very early on and often without much time for a hardened thought process, primarily because we wanted to at least be together for some period of time, even if only a short time.

June was working full time right out of high school and we were engaged a few months after her graduating. I was working two part time jobs and struggling with school, but spent every spare hour with June, knowing that I would most likely be drafted, as the war was expending and requiring more and more bodies every month. She was 19 when we married, in between my training classes and fifteen months later, was flying by herself to Hawaii to meet me on R & R, still not yet 21, then back across the Pacific and the continent to work, while living with my parents. That entire time, we had spent 1 ½ days on our honeymoon, then three months separated again while I was in NCO school, followed by three months together in Georgia as I completed my NCO on the job training. That was it until, Hawaii and the much needed R & R for the two newly weds, which would have to last us another two months. We were finally together again for the duration and looking forward to adjusting to a whole new world that we weren't really ready for, but didn't yet realize.

I have always had a whole lot of love and respect for her, the way she managed to conduct herself during those early years and continued after that rough beginning. She was a dynamo at work and excelled at anything she was given, and we began to make our way into life as a man and wife team, in hopes of having, a healthy family, and happy home for ourselves. She was also beautiful, personable, quick witted and very intelligent and more often than not, defeated me in the popular board games of the times. When playing Trivial Pursuit, my saving graces being the fact of her never caring much about sports, science and history categories, allowed me to sneak by her on a limited number of occasions. She beat me seven to eight out of ten times in most games, especially Scrabble, where being an avid reader proved a valuable aide to her and my albatross.

I spent my whole career, varied as it was, working with and training people, mostly younger, to be the best people they could be by applying what I had learned in sports, the service, from my family, friends and employers, as well as employees and customers alike. I had the good fortune to have mentors at every step of the way and always wanted to be able to pass on what I had learned, by effectively communicating well with every person I worked with, up, down and across, so they could achieve the results we all desired.

I have many friends from all of those arenas and it was always my goal to be an individual they could look up to and learn from, as to what it takes to be a good person and associate with, and develop values of fairness, honesty, equality, and integrity. After all, our integrity and reputation are the most important things we leave this life with as a good memory to others, along with, life insurance, debts and in my case, lots of stuff to sort through! I always tried to hold my temper, avoid using foul language (some crude manly examples do haunt me, but not with women or children in ear shot), and use good manners and patience with everyone, which may have been the hardest of all.

Sure, there are those who can dispel those illusions, but I'm hoping that my family will not rat me out, at least for a long while. I can truly say, that there aren't too many people, other than the mentioned family members, who can say they have seen me really mad, to the point of losing my temper. It was a red line I always wanted to draw for myself and try not cross. Unfortunately, at times, familial situations can make those lines a little fuzzy, or disappear completely.

The point I'm trying to make, is that self control is one of the best attributes a person can have, and a great tool in working to train and develop people that you want to be able to step into your job one day, if and when you retire or possibly get slapped in the face by one of your, "life's surprise attacks".

SECTION I: AMBUSH BY AGENT ORANGE

With that as a brief backdrop of that part of my personality, I'll skip to four years earlier than this writing, in my life to April, 2008. At June's insistence, she drove me to the emergency room around 1:00 AM with a blood pressure of 250 over 150 and a screaming migraine headache which I had been very accustomed to since college days. The blood pressure, though mine normally high, was much too high to avoid doing something immediately. I was, at the time, taking prescribed medication for the high blood pressure and an enlarged prostrate for the past few years, which had helped in stabilizing both conditions for the short term, but not improving it. I wasn't given a bed in the ER until several hours later at June's insistence, the admitting nurse finally found a space and admitted me.

After several days in the hospital and many lab tests and specialist consultations, I had received little relief from the headache, nor poor feeling, while accompanied by June, our children Shannon and Chris and my Mom kept a vigil. It began to become clear there was a major problem with my health and there wasn't going to be a quick fix or a fix at all, for that matter. When my kidney biopsy results came back after a few more days, we found that I had a rare disease called Light Chain Deposition Disease and it was poisoning my kidneys and my body in conjunction with my enlarged prostate which was causing my bladder to retain urine excessively. I also had up to a dozen lesions and fractures in my vertebrae, ribs, shoulder blade, neck, arm, etc. being caused by the non-curable blood cancer Multiple Myeloma. Of course we had never heard of either of these diseases and began doing as much research as possible to understand what were we're dealing with. There wasn't a lot of documentation to find at that time and not many people we talked to in the hospital had any detailed knowledge, nor had most even heard of them, so we began gathering everything we could find.

I had actually cracked several ribs while working with a work related installation crew, replacing damaged windows in early February that winter. I slipped on a patch of ice, didn't fall, but twisted my torso, luckily because there were two of us carrying the double window. We quickly sat the window down, because I knew I had at a minimum, pulled something, but when I bent down, I felt a sharp pain and couldn't take a breath. I knew that I had cracked at least one rib as I had cracked three in a HS football practice, and knew what it felt like. That ended my physical assisting for the day, but I continued coordinating and conversing with the crew, homeowner and homebuilder. I never told June, nor anyone else about the incident, just pampered myself until I was better.

A month or so later, while preparing for my first lawn cutting of the season, I realized that my mower deck had slipped loose from its mounting, so I shut it down and tried to muscle it back in place while positioning myself on the ground and trying to push and steady it well enough to hook it back up. All of a sudden I heard a loud crack, that sounded like a stick breaking. After cursing very loudly, I jumped up and paced in a big circle around the yard until the pain eased, then went to the shed and grabbed a large pry bar, which I should have done first thing. I had to change my position totally because I had to use my left arm, but finally got it repaired, and cut the grass.

I never told any one about that either, but now a month later, the fractured scapula showed up with several cracked ribs on the hospital X-rays. I explained to the doctor that I knew when and how those happened, but couldn't recall anything else, unless they might be old injuries. He told me that those were definitely fractures, and probably some of the vertebrae were, and felt that they were all most likely progression of the lesions caused by the Multiple Myeloma.

My kidneys seemed to be the largest concern for me because I was in an advanced stage on chronic kidney disease, as a result of the MM and LCDD, and bordering on having to undergo dialysis which I had no desire to take part in, because of personal experiences with the process of family and friends. The cancer was secondary in my thoughts because I believe that the mind is a large part of fighting cancer, as my mom had proven to me over the last twenty plus years, and I thought I had the positive mind set to deal with that.

We got underway immediately with chemo in the form of Velcade and Prednisone to begin the ultimate battle with cancer. Pamidronate was also prescribed to counter the bone loss caused by the Multiple Myeloma. I was doing three week chemo cycles at first, three days per week and then one week off. Those cycles continued for seven or eight months until I began the reclamation of my stem cells for the upcoming stem cell transplant.
Chemo in one form or another continued until I requested to stop them eight years later.

Lying in bed alone in the hospital at nights during that first week or so, while things were being assimilated and sinking into my brain, is about the only time I felt sad, scared and sorry for myself, just as I had felt many times before, in Vietnam and as early as basic training. I can remember laying in the bed late at night, alone and sniffling about what was ahead, but felt like I would do OK with June's love and support.

As soon as I came home from the hospital, I started back to work on a part time basis while continuing my chemo

infusions and slogging to work afterwards, and continuing the research.
Our son Chris found a tidbit of information on the internet about Multiple Myeloma having a direct association with Agent Orange, and it had just recently been approved for VA benefits,
which prompted my making an appointment with the Veteran's Administration. My Agent Orange Ambush!

I encountered several difficult setbacks in the beginning of my treatment, all a result of excessive chemo and steroids and resulted in two additional life-threatening hospitalizations of a bleeding intestinal ulcer that required emergency surgery and seven units of blood and a deep vein thrombosis respectively, followed by a bout with shingles covering my neck, head and face, right side. In addition, when I transferred my care to the VA, during an introductory dental exam, they discovered that I had osteonecrosis to my right jaw and needed immediate surgery. The osteonecrosis was caused by excessive treatments also, and I completed the surgery without complications, however I had a recurrence the following year, which was contained.

Armed with all of my medical information and discharge papers from the army, I applied for and within a few months, received approval from the VA for the accepted diagnosis of an Agent Orange/Vietnam service associated disease, Multiple Myeloma. I was barely able to stay awake and keep my head upright without partially laying my head on the desk. June kept talking to me and nudging until the counselor came in, and continued the prodding while the meeting progressed.

Having that comfort level of financial and medical coverage, I continued my fighting back. Maybe because I felt that this would not have happened to me if I hadn't been in Vietnam, maybe because it just gave me something to be mad about, or just my optimistic views. Whatever it was, it worked, because I've never looked back and felt sorry for myself for contracting the diseases. For several weeks following my release from the initial hospital stay, I had to insert catheters four to six times daily to make sure I was removing the stagnant urine, until I could be scheduled for a laser trimming of the prostate. I surely have` felt sorry for myself for other struggles I've faced since then, but not my illness.

I am not afraid that THE TIME will come before I am ready, because I have been ready and know it is coming. I won't suffer, because that is all used up and gone. I try not to complain to others about pain or how I feel, thereby pulling them into the mix, because I don't want to have anyone "suffer" along with me as we all compassionately tend to do. People always mean well, but too much empathy and/or sympathy is trying and responses become difficult. I probably lean too much in that direction when trying to console others, or fend off the concern for me and apologize for that, but I would rather that outcome that to be too much for them to bare.

I just try to move forward to get better, or at least hold my own against this incurable disease, as actually getting better or even feeling better is an up and down and sometimes daily occurrence. Three things I remember most during my consultations, Multiple Myeloma patient/caregiver group meetings and treatments over the first few months of diagnosis: 1) there is no cure, but new drugs are being discovered on a continuing basis, some with good results and more time may be added to my life expectancy if I qualified for a stem cell transplant; 2) remissions are achievable, but are not permanent, MM will always return as there is no complete remission; 3) I was told by the VA counselor that helped me with the paperwork in the beginning, as her final comment to June and I, "I can promise you one thing...when you die, MM will be the cause of your death."

Those three factors are stuck in the front of my mind and have been fortified by my readings and research and the loss of a close family friend undergoing her second stem cell transplant, part of the preferred tandem transplant. She was about eight years younger than me, and underwent her second transplant, within weeks of my first. We had talked between her's ending and mine beginning, and she offered me a great deal of encouragement about the procedure, letting me know she would be starting her second within weeks of my first and we could talk some more. Jane died of complications of MM leading to pneumonia, as her body's immunization system was nonexistent at that point in the procedure. She left a young daughter, husband, brother, mother and father, the father dying several months later, all being friends of the family since my earlier years in Georgia. Because of that and the fact that my first transplant was not fully successful, I opted not to continue with the tandem portion of that procedure and went back onto the chemo infusions once my immune system and body recuperated sufficiently.

In an odd way, I like knowing what to expect and feel that I can mentally help myself through the fight. Better than not knowing what may happen or being told everything will be OK, which is very difficult to believe when presented with a cancer diagnosis of any sort, let alone one that is not curable.

How many of us have lost loved ones without any notice or warning? I suspect we all have. To know the end is coming and why, is somewhat comforting to me because I can try in earnest to accomplish those things I want to accomplish and prioritize, while paying as much attention to family and friends as possible. As the diseases continued to take their toll, I began to realize that I couldn't even maintain a part time schedule at work and fulfill my obligations to the company, so retired shortly after my 62nd birthday and applied for early social security disability benefits. The company employees and my boss had been exceptionally gracious and lenient with me throughout the entire sequence of events, of which I am very grateful.

Not having to report to a job daily and being able to concentrate on work I wanted to get completed around our house, my Mom's house and to do things for and with my kids and grandchildren was wonderful. I was able to spend more time with my grandkids than most grandparents and enjoyed it greatly. My professional career was very rewarding, enjoyable and memorable, and I do miss the social contact that is gone, but it has been much better with no pressure to get personal things accomplished by a certain time or date, and I continue to keep in touch with friends. I built some wonderful friendships over the years at work and was extremely fortunate to work with some of the best and most professional people in the business.

I was originally diagnosed with as little as, months to a few years, as a result of my kidney damage, however they improved enough over several months, to my Nephrologists' surprise, to keep me away from dialysis, at least for the interim. My outlook improved enough for a stem cell transplant after six months which pulled me back out of my part time work for another three weeks.

As stated previously, I worked for another six months off and on after my stem cell transplant and then retired and planned a family trip to Disney World, probably to be our last as a complete family. We had a great vacation including a swim with dolphins and I continued my chemo and tinkered around the house, but didn't accomplish much as things seemed to stagnate and not get any better, but more importantly, not worse either.

Mom continued to fail as time went on and June took care of most of her needs at that time. I had to stop her from driving much to her dismay, because she was just not responsive enough, reacted too slowly, and her argument that DMV had reissued her license because she passed the eye test qualified her to drive, just wasn't sufficient.

The next few years were difficult and slow for me, in that I didn't have much energy and didn't get out much except to visit the hospital for my checkups and chemo sessions while trying to help June with Mom's needs and visiting with our family.

The months continued to pass slowly and the progress was slower, but at least things weren't getting worse for me. My grandsons did most of my outside work, as I even had a hard time riding the tractor around the yard without getting dizzy, but life moved on.

There was a somewhat complacent feeling beginning to develop within me that I was not at all comfortable with. I did not like feeling as helpless and weak as I was feeling and having to be so dependent on June fussing over me and taking care of me. I liked her attention, but having my Mom and myself to oversee was beginning to be incredibly difficult for her to manage and she was beginning to seem somewhat worn down at times.

Her "mild" lupus seemed more bothersome and was causing more visits to the specialist with more prescriptions being written, which June did not like having to take. One thing led to the other, including a few issues with lung infections and she was back and forth on doctor visits which involved me doing more for myself and Mom.

SECTION II: AMBUSH BY CANCER

The worst time in my life began about a year and half later, June was diagnosed with stage IV breast cancer while being treated for mild lupus and slight lung problems. She had continually complained of a distinct pain through two mammographies which did not produce any positive results, but while reading the chest X-rays for her lung problem, the radiologist alertly noticed the tumor in her breast.

We scheduled her appointment with her surgeon immediately and a few weeks later she had a single mastectomy which resulted in a stage IV classification because of the position of the tumor and the involvement of 23 of the 25 lymph nodes tested. A few weeks later she had a second surgery as it was determined that the first had not removed enough of the tissue within the margin required.

I accompanied June on her chemo sessions as she had with me before I transferred to the VA facility. I had to spend all day there and we chose for her not to travel with me on the two hour round trip. Her sessions were local, although covered under the VA and I always went unless I had a session on the same day. We continued in this fashion for months until she had finished her chemo and began her radiation treatments, which were also local. I chose to decline radiation on my hips because of the required daily drive to and from Philadelphia for four consecutive weeks.

June was doing as well as could be expected, other than suffering with the loss of her hair, so Chris shaved her head and we acquired a few wigs that made the loss almost unnoticeable and we were assured that she was on a path to recovery.

After the radiation treatments, we were expecting the beginning of a return to somewhat normalcy, but that never really came. She was suffering with anemia and had to have frequent blood transfusions and following further testing at Penn Cancer Center, we found that she had contracted myelodisplasia leukemia from her primary breast cancer chemo Doxorubicin, the infamous Red Devil, which I feel, all who are prescribed should think more than twice before taking.

She soon began chemo treatments for the myelodisplasia while being cross matched for amicable stem cells. Her sister had offered but was not a match and she could not use her own like I did because of her unique cancer. She had begun suffering from horrible headaches, nausea and spells of passing out. Luckily, the passing out and related falls only happened at times when I was with her and she only received a scuffed knee one time. Ambush of my Wife by Cancer and chemo!

She was my rock, my caregiver and my mom's caregiver. I was shocked and furious at the same time because it just wasn't fair. She never complained, pitied herself, or threw in the towel, but kept plugging on with as much of a smile that she could manage. She offered encouragement to others and pushed away the sympathy by acting like it was tolerable, but it really wasn't.

Several more ER visits occurred the next couple of weeks until she was again admitted and given three consecutive spinal taps looking for signs of brain cancer, however we weren't told that. When they could not determine what was causing the passing out, vomiting and low blood counts, they moved her to Penn Cancer Center in Philadelphia, where I visited her the next morning.

I met with two doctors who matter of factly explained her condition as they had taken a triple size sample with another major spinal tap and found that the cancer had metastasized to her brain liner fluid and spinal fluid. The Neoplastic meningitis was terminal, with average life time of four months, if caught early enough. Her's was not and she was diagnosed with only fourteen days to live and died at home exactly fourteen days later.

There were experimental chemo shots that were injected right into the brain stem that had shown a little success, if caught early, but were very painful and had strong side effects. I knew June could not and would not want that, as she had mentioned in the car on the way to the hospital that she wasn't going to do any thing else if it was deemed necessary, as she was too tired and weak. We had discussed that more than once for both of us and had jointly decided there came a time when enough was enough for each of us and each would decide. Shannon and Kyle were with me and I asked if the doctors would come back after we got ourselves composed and inform June of the situation including the prescribed treatment, but leaving out the worst details, and they agreed and we assembled in her room about an hour later.

After the doctors met with June and explained her situation and condition, she let them leave the room, as we were both tearing up, she hugged and kissed me and told me that she guessed I really did love her because she never thought I would take care of her like I did. I don't know why she said that. I told her that she could never know how much I loved her and always had and was so very sorry that we ended up in the position we had and reminded her that we had both promised to always take care of each other to the end.

I would not allow the doctors to tell her that she only had such a short time or that the condition was terminal, but she seemed to inherently know most of that before the talk. She had tremendous foresight and an uncanny sense of many things, including what I was thinking on many occasion, as I did with her.

We spent a few more hours with her as she was scheduled to be taken home by ambulance the next morning, to allow Hospice to get involved in her care with one daily visit and nurse on call. I ordered a hospital bed and had everything set up when she arrived the next morning and the entire family gathered and stayed continually until she passed on a Wednesday morning after a long hard night of deep and labored breathing with me sitting beside her and holding her hand.

The entire family had spent the entire time in our house for thirteen days 24/7 with only moments away for refreshed clothing. Shannon slept on the couch, Chris on the floor by the bed with Maggie under the bed by him, and me in a chair pulled up to the bed. That morning Shannon, Kameron, Kyle and I were there as the others were freshening up.

June and I had been back and forth for a little over four years at this point, with her initially being my caregiver full time while going through my operations and therapy, and then reversing things when she began her ordeal. We often altered those primary positions too, as one would feel stronger, or the other was having a rough day.
It's difficult to explain what was running through my mind during this time frame and I can't even guess everything June was thinking and feeling because she would drift in

and out of lucidity without any notice, once right in the middle of her doctor's parking lot on hot July afternoon. When she started to fall, I barely caught her in time and propped her against my bent knee for about ten minutes until it passed. A lot of love was shared between us, but it was mostly silent and just took place like it should, with no complaints coming from either side, all of which reminds me of a cute little story, or two, ok, three.

With the whole family gathered at home and minor comings and goings, we didn't get much alone time, but we did get several close moments together before she lost consciousness. The most memorable to me while we were alone as everyone ran home to change, and I had just changed her sheets and helped her into one of my big t shirts cut down the back. She was in the hospital bed in our sunroom in front of our big TV with the summer olympics entertaining us, and her favorite framed picture of a sandy beach scene and snow fence given to her a few months earlier on her birthday by her Sissy, Mary Jane and niece Sheri, hanging where she could easily see it, over the fireplace.
A very relaxing and comforting location and position for her with the cathedral ceiling and floor to ceiling windows to let the bright sunshine into the room.

I sat down beside her and realized she had slipped down too far when we had her in the sitting position, and I couldn't get her moved toward the top of the bed by myself. Upset by this, I climbed onto the bed with her, as she looked up at me like I was nuts. Straddling her on my hands and knees I told her to lock her arms behind my neck, my head between her inside elbows, while I crawled us both forward to the top of the bed using my whole body with every ounce of strength I had. Which wasn't much as I didn't and don't have much strength any longer, but that was the only way I could move her toward the head of the bed alone. We must have looked like two affection starved old has-beens or a possum mom and baby clinging underneath, and we both started laughing as I struggled moving us bit by bit. When I got her to the top of the bed, beginning to huff and puff a bit, she had repositioned her hands around my neck and was acting like she was choking me, looking at me with her funny face and her tongue sticking out at me.

I have several favorite pictures of her posing just like that when we were dating and enjoy them often, as they are positioned around the house and on my phone and computer. They are some of my favorite pictures of her, but not quite the favorites and she hadn't done that in over 40 years. The pictures of her in her bathing suit of when we were engaged and the one of us together in Hawaii on my R & R are my favorites. We both laughed and then cried until she drifted off to sleep for a nap.

Another time she wanted lotion rubbed on her feet, so I did it, as usual, with a lot of love until she gently kicked me away, and another when I was sweetly rubbing her leg until she nonchalantly lifted my hand and placed it on the bed beside her, while placing her hands crossed across her stomach, her favorite resting position in the bed. Just like it was nothing different than normal, but she was only days away from unconsciousness! My amazing wife!

I had lost my wife of 42 years, my Junie, at age 62. Now I began feeling sorry for myself, I was not going to get her back this time, and it was by far, the worst feeling of my life and put Vietnam in the far back of my head again, in proper perspective.
It remains to this day to be the most bitter period of my life and will be on the day I die.

Having lost our third family puppy a decade earlier, June and I had discussed prior to her diagnosis, that another Sheltie would be good company for her after I passed, as I had a short life expectancy. Fate totally turned that plan around and Maggie has been my 24/7 buddy ever since. June got to help train her and loved her sleeping on the bed with us. Every night when I went to bed I put Maggie up and gave her a play sock and she dropped it right in June's face, without fail every night. She hated it, but loved it at the same time and was able to get back to sleep after tossing it to Maggie a few more times. I don't know what I would have done if I didn't have Maggie's company these long, lonely years. Maggie never slept on the bed again after June was gone and had no desire to even get up there again. Neither of us sleep in our old bedroom now.

These thoughts and connecting them back with our life is all new to me, and requires new thinking because I lost her so suddenly, at least that is all that makes sense to me now. I wish I could erase all of the bad times but that is impossible and it is probably better to remember that we made the best out of those too. I can only regret that I caused those hard times, but rejoice in the fact that June had enough love for me and us and our family, to allow us to try and fix them. She could have, and maybe should have left me many times.

I could have made her life much easier had I been more open to listening to her and allowed her to help me from the beginning. I'm hearing her loudly and clearly now as I am always asking for her help with everything that gets me down and helping me find misplaced things, just like we used to do equally for each other. Whenever I cant find something now, I just pause, ask June, and I seem to automatically go to it. We always had a knack for finding what the other one lost, but not what we lost ourselves. Many situations occur like that now which bring back memories, visions, smells and touches from her which frequent my life very lovingly and thought provokingly.

Telling June that I loved her, or anyone for that matter, has been hard for me for many years now. Those three little words used to mean everything to me, and I told her so often I got on her nerves, but something changed and it became very difficult to say them. Oh, I could say luv ya, like everyone says dozens of times per day, but struggled with the three heart felt words, and that seems to me to be almost a common exchange between friends, not lovers and all very common today. I love you seems less used, maybe because of the modern methods of abbreviated communication.

I digress, sorry, I now know it to be a fairly common trait for Vietnam Veterans, and maybe a cop out. Lots of opinions why, but none I have grown comfortable with other than not wanting to express any signs of personal commitment since returning because of the loneliness and distressing events over there.

That is also one of the biggest regrets of my life and it is unbelievable how many times I said it those last months and since, throughout the days and nights when I think about her and talk to her.

June had a sense long before she was even diagnosed that she would go before me. After I got sick we talked about how she felt occasionally, and she continued to have bad feelings and I would always say she was nuts. After she was diagnosed her comments came more often and soundly, and she casually joked that it would still be so and that my Mom would probably outlast both of us. I did have a slight chuckle about that, but knowing Mom's strength in fighting cancer I agreed it could definitely happen.

I did my best to convince her that wasn't the case as Multiple Myeloma is not curable and we had been told there was a good chance of her becoming cancer free, in the beginning, before the problems. She never bought into that argument and must have had reason for feeling that way, but she never let on to anyone else about it, nor did I.

In truth, I believe both of us wanted to be the first to go. She told me that she wanted me to find someone else and I told her no way, never happen, and contrarily told her I didn't want her to find anyone else because I was too selfish and jealous, and couldn't stand the thought. I don't think either of us wanted to be here without the other. I know for sure that I felt that way and I felt June would have handled it much better than I.

What kept both of us going and is still true for me, is that we had a very strong desire for our grandchildren to remember us. At that time, the youngest was Christopher (Buddy), Chris and Angelica's son. When I was diagnosed a few years earlier, it was Kenzie, Shannon and Johnie's daughter. Now we have two more, Shannon and Von's son Max and Chris and Angelica's daughter Adriana. Kyle, Kameron, Isela and Kenzie do remember her. Buddy, Max and Adriana will unfortunately for them, not, but I still have her picture all over the house for them to see and ask questions about and we talk about her often.

I have a few more years to go, in order to ensure that Max and Adriana remember us, especially me, and I have a good start because I try to pester and tease them as much as possible, as their Bubby is well known for. We recently had to explain to Buddy that I was indeed married, to MomMom June, because he asked why I was not married, and lived alone one evening, out of the blue.

I did my best to go from patient to caregiver for June and Mom, but know I wasn't as successful as I should have been able to be. I will always regret that very much. My Mother and I developed an almost confrontational relationship in her waning years as the offspring had become the parent, a very common occurrence, I'm told. It wasn't comfortable for either of us, but that is the way it was. I will always regret that also. Mom passed about two years later giving up on her third life taking battle with cancer on December 26, 2014. She suffered from breast cancer in the eighties, colon cancer diagnosed several days after my brother Lee died of a heart attack in 1991 and finally several operations with facial melanoma and COPD.

My Dad died of a major heart attack on March 10, 1999 still grieving badly for my brother and spending most of his time in quiet solitude, away from all of us. Mom had continued to live in her new home near the rest of the family, after recently moving from our pre college time home an hour away. June and I, Shannon and Chris assisting her with shopping, transportation, medications, doctor visits, and laundry. Her great grandsons, Kyle and Kam took care of her vacuuming and yard work, and she was frequently visited by all of her great grandkids, sister and several church members.

I spent my entire time in Vietnam thinking I wouldn't see June again. Either I wouldn't make it home, or worse for me, that she would find someone else while I was away. It had nothing to do with me not trusting her, or her sending signals to that effect, but the fact that so many guys received that dreaded "Dear John" letter, that it freaked out the married men or men with a sweetheart back home. There were many young men receiving those letters during my service time and it began wearing on me early on in training because I had a sweetheart at home and a wife by the time I shipped out for Nam. In matters of the heart I guess I'm not so perfectly optimistic, in fact, seemingly very pessimistic and fearful.

While training and learning to march, the drill sergeants often called cadence, as all units do, and chanted cadence songs involving "Jody", the alias for every nasty woman stealer in The World (GI's acronym for the USA/home). The storied "Jody" ravaged any lonely and weak lovers or wives of soldiers away from home, and especially in Vietnam. There were many crude choruses which depicted the ugly scenes, and while seemingly humorous to listeners, as trite as it might seem, it became a reality as the men began receiving their letters as early as basic training with increasing regularity, as their tours continued. By the time we were still FNG's (Fucking New Guy) in Vietnam, they became all too frequent and created some nasty displays of fighting, searches for the Padre, self-inflicted wounds and even suicides.

I spent two years in ROTC at U of D learning basic military tactics, weaponry, etc., but mostly drill and ceremony. However, we never had those types of cadences called while marching, only those that promoted unit prowess, cadences chanted to challenge other units on the parade grounds around the world and more importantly, morale builders. I guess certain things affect certain minds in different ways, and it definitely added a major concern for me. I truly dreaded the thought and would reread letters from June to look for between the lines clues that something was coming. Yes, I felt guilty for that and I still do, but I was scared. For many, the favorite activity of mail call, became an anxiety of mixed feelings at times. I am not putting myself in that category because June did nothing to make that a possibility for me, but the proof of others who did was all around me. My guess is that most of the "lifer" drill sergeants had received or had friends that received those letters during their tours were trying to prepare the newbies for reality. If you expect it, it won't hurt so bad. Wrong!

I wrote as often as possible to June and every few weeks to my parents and grandmothers, less often to my brother and friends. I would write ahead several letters to June and stagger their mailing because I couldn't always write daily. That strategy was suggested to us while processing into country by a wise E-8 (MasterSergeant). He also suggested we keep everything bland and non threatening as well as sanitized about locations and activity, in order to keep our family less worried when watching the ever present evening news and reading the newspaper, as well as for security. I did that without fail except to my best friend Mel, who I swore to secrecy. No need to create more worry than necessary, as their waiting and loneliness had to be every bit as intimidating as ours or maybe even worse.

My Mom once told me many years later, that it was the hardest thing she had ever gone through, bar none. This from a woman who's husband flew all over the world during WW II, lost one of younger twin brothers at 19 of a heart defect, the other a few years later in the Pacific war as a pilot, a seven year old sister from diphtheria, her oldest son at age 45 and had fought through two serious operations, chemo and radiation treatments for cancer.

Others wrote very colorful and often obscene descriptions of what was happening, including photographs of same, many, very X-rated, showing mutilated bodies, even though we were warned of letters and especially photographs, being opened and censored.

I believe that training films and all of the, probably exaggerated information, war stories, etc. of VD and what prostitution techniques in country did to us young men, to be some of the most important training we received. No one with common sense or any sense at all, would seek a prostitute after seeing some of those training films of the "black crud", blue balls, extreme syphilis, white cong, or even basic crabs. Right? Unfortunately the answer is Wrong. Statistically, approximately one in four Vietnam Veterans were diagnosed with VD while in country. Totally disgusting, not to mention crossed razor blades used by prostitutes. How about that ice cold coke loaded with ground glass for a departing gift, or heroin laced marijuana? No thanks, and for me at least, absolutely no chance! Those training aids, to me, were right up there with how to clean and care for your weapons. The training media, and "Jody" cadences resounded strongly with me for my entire tour and I took as few chances possible, with anything I had been warned about. I wish that many more had taken notice and I hope the military still pushes the former, but uses the more benign cadence songs relating to the attributes of unit histories to build spirit and cohesiveness.

My anticipated R & R (Rest & Recuperation) is what kept me going for my first seven months in country. Everyone was entitled a one week leave to a list of destinations after three months in country, one per tour. Honolulu was the designated choice for those who were married and could afford flying their spouse and wanted to meet their spouse in that paradise. Single men had the option of Thailand, Australia, Japan, Hong Kong, Singapore, Seoul, Manila, etc, where the military had arranged for relaxing adventures for the lonely GI. Some of the stories of the wonderful times enjoyed by soldiers, were so enticing, it caused some married men to opt for that instead of bringing their loved ones to Hawaii, go figure. Counting down the days to meet June in Hawaii was key to keeping a good attitude for me and after returning from R & R, looking forward to being closer to going home, a short timer, soon to be an ex soldier and in her arms.

Most soldiers started a 365 count off shortly after arriving in country, ranging from simple number count-offs on helmet covers, to elaborate depictions of both sordid and patriotic images divided like a 365 piece puzzle. Each puzzle piece numbered sequentially around the images in a target scheme, to the center "#1", where you would have completely colored in each day when the image was finished. Most were the promiscuous type and you can use your imagination of where the last day of a pictorial centerfold, was indicated, so I don't have to be vulgarly descriptive.

The patriotic usually a flag, a dead gook, or maybe a weapon or freedom bird, all boring by comparison, and rarely used. Home state flags were also very popular wall decorations in private bunk areas in stand down hooches and usually the only decoration other than your personal weapon hanging on the wall. It was common knowledge that a GI could request a free flag from their home state by requesting one via mail from state capitals. Of course I had my state flag, M-16 and picture of June in her bathing suit.

How short are you, was the common question from short timer to FNG from day 365? It was usually encountered those first few minutes as those leaving country were standing by to replace the seats on the freedom bird that you just arrived in, as you and your buddies vacated. The stares in those soldiers' faces, especially the eyes, was almost scary and what was soon to be known as the thousand yard stare, blank, non-feeling, non-caring, cold stare. The very look of isolation and despair of all hope lost, even though they were on their way home. And if you took the time to glance around, you would notice pallets of silver coffins waiting to be loaded into the next available stateside bound jet.

The response to how short are you, was a slow and disgusted three digit number shout. Mid tour GI's might ask short timers, how short are you and the number would be shouted out more matter of factly, the lower it became. Two digit midgets boastfully shouted out "99 short" on that memorable morning and would now start announcing more frequently with increased joy as the days passed. The "short!" announcements became daily and more automatic and forceful at 30 days short, even without the prompting of a question, until it got to single digits and 5,4,3, and "2 and a wake up", or "I'm so short I could sit on a penny", or "I have to sleep on the floor", or "I could milk a cow without a stool", or "I can't reach the piss tubes" (plastic drain pipe inserted into the ground for urination), etc, etc, etc.

Toward the end of the occupation, starting in 1971, you could blow those digits away by obtaining an early out, and you would end up with less than three months remaining in your tenure with the Army. Early outs might be granted for family hardships, employment opportunities, attending college, etc. I applied for and was granted a ninety day drop for returning to college. I had to obtain acceptance from the university, have my family research courses, semester starting dates, my accrued credits record, etc. I still have the letter I wrote and typed and stenciled for dozens of copies to my commanding officer, et.all. I was granted that early out and arrived home after nine months in country and only two months following my R&R with June. It was the best correspondence I ever produced, before and after, and the timing luckily coordinated with a combat unit relocation reassignment I volunteered for prior to it being approved, as well as the start of summer classes.

I had been to Honolulu twice with my father in 1965 between tenth and eleventh grade on two of his flights and fell in love with Hawaii and a stewardess for a week (in my mind). My R & R (Rest & Recuperation) was June's only trip and we had planned to spend our time sightseeing, me staring at June, beach combing, flushing the toilet, eating, me staring at June, shopping, flushing the toilets, showering and staring at June, all very rare experiences for me the last seven months. Get the picture?

She was waiting for me with the other spouses at the R&R center and after an exciting and lengthy greeting, we strolled outside in the beautiful weather and took a cab to our hotel right off of Waikiki beach by the International Market Place. I couldn't believe how pretty she was, and pale and she couldn't believe how dark and thin I was. I showered and shaved and flushed the toilet a dozen times just because I could, and we visited a few local shops to outfit ourselves like tourists with tropical flowered shorts, shirts, shifts, bathing suits and hats. We stopped back in the room to change, and headed directly, almost directly, to maybe the most famous and beautiful beaches in the world. I warned her about the sun, but she managed a mild burn in under an hour anyway, and suffered the entire week, but not to the point of missing out on a thing. For her it was the beginning of her Spring, for me I had been in 90-110 degree weather with full bore sunshine for months after the monsoon season.

We filled our days between visiting the well known tourist sites and enjoying the beaches during the day and luaus and Hawaiian nightclubs and again the beaches at night. It was the fastest and best week in my life and I had to leave her back at the terminal, waiting for her flight, while I climbed aboard my plane with 200 plus other teary eyed, depressed soldiers that were tempted to go AWOL (Absent

With Out Leave) in lieu of returning to the war. What a choice Uncle Sam had dumped on in our collective laps.

June and I vowed to get back there later in life and finally, actually did make the plans with our reservations set a few months ahead for the winter 2002, for our thirty-second anniversary. We never did go because, when the time came, it was only months after 9/11, and we didn't feel comfortable enough with air travel to make the long trip and cancelled. We decided to postpone it until I retired, but the trip never happened because of our illnesses. My Mom and Dad had gone there on their 25th wedding anniversary two years before I went to Vietnam, and we thought it a nice idea to try to duplicate, but Chris was in his Junior year of high school wrestling on our 25th.

I don't have very much recollection of my time in country after R & R, or right before. Probably some selective memory and have discussed it with my counselor, who advised me of the possibility of regressive hypnosis in an attempt to restore the memories, but I have no real desire to engage in that. I don't even remember getting back off the plane in Vietnam, nor how I got back to my unit, but remember everything about Hawaii from the moment I saw June standing with a yellow and green flower lei around her neck, green, blue and white sun dress, crafted by my mom, and white sandals, to the time when I got back on my plane. I do have very vivid memories of everything prior to that from my stepping off the plane from the states up to my temporary assignment and first few days of it, then memories start to scatter.

I do know I made it back from Vietnam because of my incredible love for June. Had I not fallen in love with her and married her before I left for overseas, I'm sure I would not have made it back. So much was my desire to be with her again, to start a family and take care of her, that it drove me to promise myself and June that I would come back to her.

I think I've always known these things, but it didn't really sink in until a few weeks after she passed. I knew I was going to have a very rough time with her not being here with me, but never had a clue as to how totally empty I feel without her. It's not that my daughter Shannon, my son Chris, their spouses and my seven grandkids (24 to 2) aren't good for me...certainly they are and I am grateful and proud of them all, but I spent forty-five years with June and totally depended on her to keep me grounded, functional and sane.

Most importantly, I knew she was my "soul mate" and that I could never replace the connection and love that we shared from the time she was 17 and I was 20 years old. I have since mentioned to several friends that you pick your friends and especially your spouse, but you don't pick your family. Your family is blood, your spouse and you create that new blood, and it requires deep trust and love to make a good life and family work.

We were introduced to each other during my freshman year in college, she being a sixteen year old sophomore in high school. A good friend of mine Jeff, was a lifeguard at the apartment complex where she lived with her sister, brother-in-law and niece, Sheri. I immediately liked the whole bunch, and Jeff and I spent a lot of time with them playing cards, board games, swimming, talking and became interested in skydiving, as her brother-in-law was an avid jumper and convinced us to try it also, so we did.

June was dating someone at the time and I was going about my bachelor routine of playing the field, flying and playing at studying, working for a security company at concerts and hotels at a local beach. I even brought back a set of drumsticks from a Herman's Hermits concert and a shirt worn by Mickey Dolenz, of the Monkees, which June wore to the beach regularly. I wasn't a very dedicated student and wasn't really very interested in college, other than hanging around with friends and trying to meet girls.

Several of my friends had joined the Air Force with a four year commitment after working for two years and I was on a college deferment after registering for the draft. I wanted to join the army and fly helicopters but my Father forbid it as long as I was living in his household. I went to the U of Delaware and lived at home because my parents wanted me to and because my brother Lee was attending also, but really had no interest in leaving my hometown or living on campus as Lee was doing. Just wanted to put my time in and take whatever came at me.

June and I grew closer as time went on but there was not a romantic connection, at least from her point of view. I was definitely interested, but didn't want to intrude on her relationship, so we just remained good friends. I did however manage to visit her while babysitting in the complex a half dozen times or so to keep her company and help with the kids.

One spring day, I got a phone call from her sister telling me that June had broken up with her boyfriend, was somewhat distraught, and wanted to know if I would ask to take her sister to her senior prom since she had already bought her dress and the tickets. I pretended to be cool and told her sister that I would certainly think about it. I soon stopped jumping up and down and patting myself on the back, and a few hours later that night, telephoned Junie and asked her to consider letting me escort her and she accepted. Shortly afterward, I invited her to go to a movie with me so we could, sort of break the dating ice before the prom came around, and in a few days we went on our first date with her niece Sheri in tow.

Junie lived with her sister Mary Jane and was Sheri's babysitter for a few years. Eight years younger than June, and a lot of fun to be around, Sheri wound up going on a lot of dates, trips to the beach and airplane rides with June and I over the next few years, as it it allowed us to date in lieu of staying home and watching Sheri. Great compromise for the three of us and we had some great dates with no third wheel syndrome.

June began working at the Memorial Hospital in Wilmington the summer she graduated and I became her chauffeur back and forth until I took her to see a high school buddy of mine and she bought a used VW bug. I taught her how to drive a stick shift and took her to get her license and she started sprouting her wings. She was an excellent employee and improved her position steadily to a Unit Manager position in charge of about one third of the hospital unit clerks.

June continued working and advancing her career position during and after my service tenure. After my tour in Vietnam, I began working at the local Chrysler assembly plant, where I had worked during the summer after graduating HS, on the assembly line and was promoted to a trainer position during my second year. June and I were expecting Shannon the following year and moved from our apartment to a new four bedroom townhouse a few miles away. We added our first Shetland sheepdog, Misty Dawn to the family slightly before Shannon arrived and continued to learn and grow as a family.

I began having some problems with depression, bad dreams, sweats, and malaise a short time later and my family doctor tried in vain to figure out the problem. I was tested for malaria to eliminate a recurrence or carryover from Vietnam, and various Chrysler related component materials for possible allergic issues, all to no avail.

June and I struggled along, being somewhat handicapped by my situation. PTSD (Post Traumatic Stress Disorder) was not recognized at that time and I had never been to a Veteran Administration hospital or doctor since my discharge from the army. We had no idea why I was the way I was, so we just started looking for things we could do to help the situation, to create a more stable and valid family life. My condition definitely caused some tension in the family, but we dealt with it as well as possible, without knowing the cause. June was having problems relating to me also, but I attribute that to my lack of affection and for her, and the normal postpartum depression, which did slightly arise again followings our son's birth four years later.

Soon after these problems began to show themselves, the economy started slowing down and the country experienced its first gas shortage, which impacted the entire auto industry. My plant was shut down for changeover and began layoffs for newer employees. My seniority wasn't in immediate jeopardy, however June and I thought that maybe a change, under the circumstances would be a thing to consider because I was working night shift at the time of shut down, as well as the possible allergy situation. I began a job search and soon was accepted by an international consulting company headquartered in Chicago. The job was Monday through Friday, but I would be working anywhere in North America and had to arrive at the job location by Sunday night. The money was much better than Chrysler, I got a per diem allowance, and an company air travel card to fly first class, and I loved flying, especially first class.

There were many long discussions between June and I and June's mother before we accepted the job. Obviously, there would be a big strain on June with me gone Sunday evening until sometime late Friday night or worse during some conditions, June having a toddler at home and a full time job with an hour drive away. Her mother agreed to stay with us and watch Shannon during the day and as needed on weekends. We decided to give it a chance, but were definitely wary of the family situation and any unseen impact on my health, which was not determined a medical problem at the time, but definitely a concern.

That next Sunday, off I went to Knoxville, Tennessee, late Sunday afternoon en route to a cow and hog slaughter house and processing plant, my worst nightmare. I had hated, and always will hate seeing animals suffer, and remembered a class trip in grade school to a Swift slaughter house in Georgia, which resulted in my being sick and not being able to get sights, smells and sounds out of my head for a long time afterwards. This job brought it all back, only 100 times worse, because I had to study and develop every job station on both kill floors as my first assignment. I did my best to compartmentalize those negative feelings, dug in, began learning the job and doing very well as I progressed through many other clients of varying industries, primarily manufacturing and scattered locations, after four months at that location

June and I were doing well, but probably not better, as it was a real struggle for us both, as to being lonely for the other and doubly hard for her having to manage everything on the home front alone. There were some good things, as the optimist and common sense drivers in me worked overtime. The most obvious and welcomed, that being together only two days a week deterred arguments, and almost eliminated them entirely. Slight arguments usually occurred over some nightly phone calls when helpless feelings surfaced from both of us because of being so far apart and my being unable to physically "fix" anything that was a nuisance at home.

June's mother was a wonderful help to both of us, physically and emotionally for June and emotionally for me knowing that she was there for June and Shannon. The downside to that, mother in daughter's domain syndrome, and parent to adult child attitudes and vice versa, however, the good heavily outweighed the bad. I had a tremendous relationship with Theresa and loved to kid around with her, and I know we would not have been nearly as successful had she not be willing to help out. I always did my best to help and watch out for her after that. She and Shannon and Chris ended up having a lasting relationship like my grandmother and I, one they will never forget.

The other good things were that I think we both appreciated what the other was doing to keep the family moving forward and finally, the financial picture was improving rapidly, which takes a lot of pressure off of other things. Not just because of the pay, but because less expense at home because shopping and entertainment trips declined, as we basically stayed at home on weekends.

And finally for me personally, I always loved seeing how beautiful June was after being away from her. My mistake, not letting her know how I felt and the lack of expressing emotions was still there and not really improving other than the steady hello and goodbye. I hate myself for not recognizing and understanding that more fully at the time, and the rest of her life. I could have made things so much better for all of us but I couldn't even forcefully make myself do it without feeling false about it, and I truly did love her as much as ever. I'm very sure that my positioning also changed hers over time subconsciously, to the point that we both expected it, but much worse, accepted it as just being that way. My fault!

Later in life I have tried to offer advise to other young couples having issues, and always point out that I firmly believe most married couples problems are primarily related to money and sex, and not talking about any and all problems, no matter what stage of marriage. It is hard for me to go back and remember differently. Couples must be able to navigate those issues with truth, openness, common solutions and resolve by communicating.

I continued to learn my new trade quickly, began to be noticed by clients from Toronto, Detroit, Georgia, New Jersey, and more importantly by my superiors. I was promoted in slightly over a year and being considered again a year and half later.

Being home only on weekends has one real good benefit. If your wife gets pregnant, you have some very valid information to feed the obstetrician's timetable for date of delivery calculations, if they want help. We did, I did, the doctor did, and Christopher, our son did arrive three weeks after predicted by the doctor, but right on schedule for the detail oriented mind, mine! The memorable date was four and half years after Shannon was born, on the date of the biggest snowstorm in ten years in Detroit, where I was currently working. I was having delay after delay getting out early on a Friday afternoon, because of the snow threat, and knowing that Chris was coming Saturday for certain because I had arranged it with June's doctor. Yes I did!

I called the doctor several days earlier as a result of June's anxious concerns, but unknown to her. The doctor had predicted a two week earlier delivery and felt that June's nerves and the anxiety associated with me traveling, and trying to hit the weekend target caused her to hold off, then tense up too much to be able to relax and slide into labor (a crude male interpretation). At least that is what I pushed for, knowing my wife's temperament, AND, the exact date of conception!!!

We agreed that Saturday would be the perfect day to induce labor and committed to see each other in a few days, barring an unexpected delivery. Finally arriving back home and finding the storm was coming with me, I pulled into the snow covered driveway of my parents' house with a big hand made sign sticking out of a snow drift, "It's a Boy, our first Grandson" that my Dad had made out a piece of plywood wrapped in plastic.

June had asked to go to their house as a safety measure because of the storm and her mother did not drive, plus my arrival time was uncertain, if at all. I did gulp at first, thinking I had missed the big event, because we didn't know what the sex was back then and wouldn't want to know, if we could have known. After two granddaughters, Shannon and Shelly, Lee's daughter, Dad was sure that their third would be a boy, in that he was an only child. Lee and I, and Mom's sisters had three sons to the older, and two sons and the very last a girl, to the younger sister. It had to be, by all logic and chance, but we would have to wait until the next day.

After saying hello to everyone and trying to get my arms around my lovely round wife, I asked her if she was ready. She of course, said she had been ready for three weeks, but didn't really feel that the time was near. I grabbed her hand, put my ear to her belly and told her that she would be in labor tomorrow, midday, to which she laughed and said, what are you talking about?

I spilled the beans and she didn't believe me. I assured her that I truly arranged it with her doctor because it was obvious that she couldn't coordinate her anxiety well enough, and had already rolled through the two previous weekends without success. I also reminded her that I knew the exact conception date and looked up the gestation days in the Detroit library and in fact, the baby was due tomorrow. She laughed and I could see the relief in her face as she just smiled and glowed.

Yes, Christopher was born the next morning, late morning, after June broke water that night. June's experience with Shannon revealed quite a long timeframe between the two events, allowing me to play a round of golf at her insistence, and Christopher (and June) followed suit.

Sunday came quickly and I was jetting back to Detroit in first class all by myself bragging and boasting as proud fathers do, sipping on my Tanqueray gin and Fresca, my standard one drink, served by the same stewardess that had been serving me for the past several weeks. It must have been one of her favorite bid trips because she didn't have to do anything after that drink, and it was ready as soon as she saw that I was on the flight again. Change of plans, that night I celebrated with a second drink and a couple bags of peanuts, the lone passenger in first class, a perk of my employer.

Almost a year later, I was working for a company in northern NJ, following weeks in Pennsylvania, Michigan, Georgia, Alabama, Florida, Nebraska, Arkansas, Texas, New York, Missouri, California, Ohio, Illinois, Minnesota, and Montreal, Toronto, and Winnipeg, not in that order. Primarily working for manufacturing and sales companies and in all facets of their operations, learning more and more.

I was an experienced manager on this NJ job, an almost 50% increase over my original pay and I was being advised by my boss that I was being considered for my next move, which was to his level, after this job or the next. June and I were very excited about that and the financial aspect of the change from Chrysler was finally seeming worth while as an offset to all of the negative points as well as seemingly easing our communication situation simply because we were settling into a pattern, with one exception. We had that new baby boy and things were getting tougher on June with going back to work after her maternity leave ended. We thought she would probably be able to quit and stay home with the kids when I achieved that next level.

Ironically, I was nearing the end of the job I was currently working in, and the superiors of that company really liked me. Summer had ended and the company's higher ups and spouses were heading to Virginia Beach for their annual business planning session and asked me to go along and assist in the planning, without my staff or superiors. It was an odd request but I didn't think anything of it and passed the request on, to attend.

My superiors thought it was odd also and asked if the client had been hinting to me about going to work for them, and I replied no. They approved the trip and reminded me that I had signed a no compete contract with the company when I signed on, and that it was iron clad and I could be sued for breech of contract should I leave. I told them I understood that and had no intention of leaving, as I was doing so well and the company had such a dynamic retirement fund, especially at the next level where I was headed.

Twenty percent of everyone's pay was matched and added into the fund, if you quit before ten years you lost everything (a high turnover job because of the travel, especially for family people, so a lot of money building quickly), plus the interest accrued. You were 100% vested after ten years and the money stayed in the total company pot until retirement continuing to grow with washouts and interest. Many people quit or got fired before vesting, and had to leave everything there and it was divided by the remaining employees. The scuttlebutt was, $1,000,000+ payout minimum, if you retired or left after that ten years, and I was at that time, just thirty-one years old. The future looked sound and prosperous, if I could last at least another seven years, much better, if lasting longer.

I flew to Virginia Beach a few weeks later as the meetings were ready to begin and was called to the first session with all of the client's midlevel management, minus spouses. That meeting was just a cocktail party and preliminary session where everyone from across the US and Canada, mingled and reintroduced themselves. The company had service and parts operations throughout North America and Central America, which had a separate meeting.

I had worked with the twelve or so managers in the states and Canada at their locations, but had not met with some of the corporate people. Toward the end of that meeting, the VP of the client company came over, leaned into me and told me he was going to hire me away from my company and smiled. I informed him of the no compete contract and he smiled again and told me he knew, and that his company lawyers had already checked and assured him that nothing could be done to me because by law, I had the right to work to put food on my family's table and besides, his parent company, a Fortune 500 company would decline any further work with my company if they fought it. With that said, he called the corporate VP of personnel over, introduced us and verified what he had told me.

Totally shocked and shaking, I told him that I would have to sell my house, had a new baby and would have to talk to my wife, who also worked, but that I had gotten a nice raise the year before and was recently told that I was up for another step up. He smiled and asked me what the step up would total out for me, which I gave him because those were fixed salaries, by position in my company. He looked at the VP personnel and threw out a number that was about $8,000 over the projected increase I gave him.

They further offered to pay a moving company to move us, including a flat 10% value of goods for damage, cover settlement on my new and existing home, 10% of salary for carpeting and drapes and a few other spiffs. I was totally shocked as he asked what I thought about the offer. "I'm definitely interested", I said and he told me to call June and get her down there the next day so she could meet he and his wife and the others and discuss the package in order to give him an answer so they could include it into the business plan.

I called June and she was shocked more than I, but very interested because it definitely seemed that she could stay home with the kids, a joint dream we both had, as I had always secretly wanted her to have the choice of a stay at home Mom from the start. I called my parents, ran through the scenario and a couple hours later, June was driving four hours at night, alone, across the Chesapeake Bay Bridge Tunnel for the first time, and by far the longest solo drive of her life. The kids snugged into beds in my parents' house, they most likely shaking their heads as if saying, what the heck just happened. I never would have expected June to commit to the whole lot, especially immediately, but she did and was really excited about it, but a very guarded excitement, I'm sure, because she was not nearly as spontaneous nor optimistic as me.

I finished the evening out with the guys getting a lot of smiles and elbow pokes as the word spread of the offer.

Most were good with it, but there a few that I had rubbed wrong (their view point, not mine) or immediately felt I was probably taking something that could be theirs. The natural jungle feelings when something like that happens within or out of an organization. When people started back to their rooms, I went back to mine, pulled out the calculator and notebook and started ciphering and trying to answer questions I anticipated from June.

Hearing a knock at the door and realizing that June was a little ahead of the schedule I had planned out for her, I opened the door, wrapped my arms around her and pulled her into the room, the pair of us with big, quizzical smiles plastered on our faces. We talked and pelted each other with questions most of the night until we passed out on the bed. It was Friday night and the meeting agenda for Saturday was open, for couples to explore as they wished, with a big dinner scheduled that night. June was as nervous as I've ever seen her, but beautiful as always. She did not like to socialize with strangers any more than I did, and she just didn't get as much exposure to it. I had met my future bosses family several times as he had invited me for dinner at his house and I thought a lot of his wife, who was born in Greer, SC, right up the road from where Mom was born, a nice southern lady and I knew she would take care of June at the dinner and help her get settled later.

June and I had come to a solid agreement to give the move and job a try. She had barely gotten back to work after maternity leave with Chris and was having some issues at work with her slightly chauvinistic boss. Timing is everything and the money was taken care of, plus more. I knew the housing was a good bit more expensive as were the taxes, but all things considered, we had decided three years earlier to keep pushing ourselves for changes in an effort to get to where we wanted to be, wherever that was, as if anyone ever knows. We had a very nice dinner and the entire ensemble headed back to the hotel walking in pairs, June and I with my new boss and wife. He had made an announcement at dinner and had introduced us to the group.

Sunday morning, June and I hopped in the car and headed back home full of hope and angst, but things worked out well and several weeks later, my new company also providing me an efficiency motel room while we searched for homes. We found and purchased a beautiful older house on a acre of land at the base of a mountain with a small lake in view from the front. My consulting company put up no fight, even brought my old bosses and current crew to a going away dinner for me, and I suspected the threat from the parent company of no future business had been issued.

The new job was going nicely, and I was given the added responsibility of reorganizing a few of the departments and given another increase about fifteen months in. The kids were growing, Shannon began school and took dance lessons and Chris stayed home with his mom. June made good friends with a couple neighbors which gave her some company during the day and we made some modifications to the house, but it was hard on her because she was used to her work routine and spending a good bit of time with her sister and Mother, which was now missing but for occasional visits back and forth.

Work kept me very busy, but we tried to get to some activities in the city, as we were about an hour northwest of New York City. One of my best friends from HS had been divorced, remarried and lived near us so we got together occasionally for dinner or a play in the city. She and June were friends also, as she and her first husband were one of our original gang of couples that always partied together after we all got married. My brother and his family lived about an hour and half west into PA, so we visited each other occasionally as well as going back home to visit both families with a two hour drive. We took a week in the summers and rented a house back at the beaches June and I haunted while dating continuing a family tradition of summer beach vacations.

Things began getting a little tense again between us as everything was moving forward and she had become bored and lonely for home. June decided she wanted to go back home with the kids and go back to work, my company had just been bought out and the first thing they did is get rid of my boss, so I started getting nervous also and began sending out resumes. I met with the VP of personnel and discussed the situation and asked if he could let me go with severance. He explained that was impossible, that I could quit or tough it out and wait for the inevitable, which I did.

We had just gone through the second fuel shortage in 1979-80 with long gas lines, the longer travel became rough for us and everyone else, so the visiting was curtailed. We continued with the ups and downs of life and we were definitely heading downward as things seemed to fester and we let them stew. We decided to do a civil divorce, but like most, it turned nasty and we fought a good bit. We finally sold the house, split down the middle and June headed back home, rented a small house by her sister and I rented an apartment near work, paid her support and began looking for a new job, anywhere. We were now in a recession 1981 and jobs were very tough to find, especially jobs like I was accustomed to. I mailed out over two hundred resumes from FL to NY and received less than a dozen replies. I knew I was going to have to start all over again, but what choices did I have.

I drove down and stayed with June and the kids every other weekend and did my thing with Shannon and Chris, maintaining a sociable relationship with June. It was very hard for me not to be able to return to her, I knew that I needed her and I was getting worse. They finally did get to me at work, but the VP of personnel made sure I received six months severance pay and gave me a written letter of reference explaining the situation, the final statement being, "The new management is struggling while bringing their own people in and all I can say, is that if they can't get along with and work with Jim, they can't get make it with anyone." That reference and several others by former consulting clients, were on every resume I printed from that point on.

Our lawyers were doing what many lawyers do, cause as many arguments as possible and create more billable hours until there is no money left. A harsh and cynical view I know, but it is how we both felt. But most likely because of me continually reluctant in showing my affection and lack of emotion, I just made things worse. We were all but wiped out and decided for the kids' sake, to squander most of what was left, in order to continue our tradition and return to the beach for our annual summer family vacation, minus two hearts. So that we did, and I rented the nicest place we had ever used, and for Shannon and Chris, we went through the motions for the seven days with June going to the bedroom while I slept on the couch after the kids went to bed. It was bitter sweet, but I was so glad we were able to accomplish the charade. We headed back north, past the point where June's VW bug had lost its engine exactly eleven years before, I dropped them off at their house and continued back to my crappy efficiency apartment.

June and I began talking almost daily after that and discussed trying to make things work again and after about five weeks of back and forth, she called one afternoon and asked what I was going to do, and that I had better "shit or get off the pot". I said give me a couple days to get things together, and she said "today". I was there within three hours, having dropped off a letter at the apartment office on my way, breaking my lease.

We had no plans, not much money and no job. I had canvassed the home turf with resumes for several months prior with negative results, but registered with a personnel agent and started again. Nothing going on in my pay category, nor anywhere close but my agent was totally in love with my experience and job history. She personally called my references and said she had never before received all references with such positive comments, and insisted I take her written notes of them with me on interviews. Everyone was impressed but I was deemed overqualified.

While at this point in my story I want to include a fact that the only mention of my army service that the professionals wanted on my resume was the years I served and my rank. They wanted it as bland as possible and I was rarely questioned about where I served and what I did unless the interviewer happened to be a veteran or maybe was a relative of one. That started at my first job, but the consulting company and my next employer were interested because they were vets and they wanted to get to know me. My next job lasted eleven years followed by a seventeen year tenure leading to my retirement and I did discuss my service there because I knew the interviewers and they were definitely interested in my entire career, to get a look at the complete picture.

It was roughly, that ten to fifteen year period, 1971-1986 when I felt that military service counted against you, especially if you served in Vietnam and were in a combat unit. Now, so many people on facebook and other social media sites are always gushing over Vietnam vets and pumping them up, posting patriotic messages, asking questions about their service and calling a lot of attention to them. I often wonder if they are those demonstrators that marched against the war, patrolled the airports looking for lone GI's to confront, and did whatever and whenever possible to disparage the veterans personally by calling them drug addicts and baby killers, etc. If it is them, is it that they are eaten up with guilt and asking for forgiveness, or just feeling sorry about it? It is one thing to dislike the government for how they run a war, or anything else for that matter, but it is just wrong to personally take it out on the soldiers, and not remember how many of them were drafted and served as well as those who enlisted for family or patriotic reasons.

They should have at least been equally vocal about those who deserted and defected rather than fight or obtain conscientious objector status and help the wounded or worked in other non combat functions. And if willing to give up your citizenship because you didn't want to go or were afraid to go, or worse desert your fellow soldiers you trained with, why accept a pardon to come back, why not stay? And if you come back, why not be made to do it as an immigrant and/or have to re-earn your citizenship that you so easily gave up?

Is it the veterans themselves seeking the attention because they got no positive recognition? If you are a vet, are you pissed that there was no recognition, you got spit at, feel ignored, feel discriminated against, condemned as a drug addict just because you were there, or the many other criticisms? You must let it go and you hopefully will begin to feel better because you can't keep dwelling on it, it's history and because of it, things improved for future soldiers. That's the facts.

You can see it with your own eyes, you can tell by my writing, I was upset about it too, but that was then and now is now, but the memories certainly do remain. While in country and after returning home, have you learned to shove things away, hide them deep in your soul, lost trust in those you loved, lost faith in government to be truthful, lost your religion, become emotionless, lost ability to show compassion, wonder when agent orange is going to sneak up on you or your offspring, became an alcoholic or drug addict and confused as to why, feel guilty that you escaped unscathed or made it home, have no place to sleep or live but the street, ache and hurt all over, think you are going crazy, continue to have nightmares, break into a sweat and become nostalgic when you hear a helicopter, especially a Huey, jump or dive when you hear an explosion, add a "fuck" to every other word when upset, pushed loved ones away or lost them entirely because any or all of these feelings and emotions!

Of course you do, are and will continue to. It never goes away fully, at least not for me. But you have to try, just as the loss of a loving spouse never goes away, in fact for me, that gets worse.

Getting very nervous day by day, following a day of appointments, June told me that her sister's husband had mentioned to his boss, the owner of a local building material company was interested in talking to me. I went over to their house and asked him a few questions, mainly what was he looking for in a new employee and he told me sales and management. June and I talked it over quickly and decided I'd better take a look at it because things weren't getting any better so I called and set up an appointment. The meeting was fine, and I liked him well enough but he had no job remotely close to matching my resume work history.

I had learned to sell myself and my companies services, but no other tangible products, other than at the hardware store during college, but he didn't seem to mind. He wanted to hire me on the premise of me learning the business at entry level income (gross was less than I had been paying in taxes), helping him hire and train new employees with the intention of his expanding and growing the company into new product areas even he was not familiar with, increasing my pay as we progressed. Maybe he had illusions of grandeur, I had no idea, but he did seem sincere and nothing else was sitting there waiting for me, so I said ok.

I, or I should say we, took it and bored ahead. We soon moved to the beach area temporarily after me getting an education in the product and company, in the hopes of building enough business down there to develop the workload of a new branch in Dover, the middle of the state. June began working for an eye doctor and made some fun, new friends, Shannon in school and Chris in daycare and I have a company car and developing new customers, scouting for new store locations, helping the young lead person in the Dover store develop into a manager. I was also commuting back up north in between everything else, to work and begin planning with my boss, the owner's son in law who was the President of the company. His wife was VP and wanted to help bring in new retail and home builder products, tear down the old and ancient store and build two new modern buildings and office spaces while refurbishing other existing buildings.

Her mother, the actual owner, was a very nice southern lady whom I got along with famously, even asked by her to introduce the guest of honor at her birthday party, to her friends, employees and family, I assumed because of my southern accent. The goal of the company was to sell products to the entire state and develop new divisions by adding new products such as kitchens, lighting, windows, doors and service of all products. By the end of the first year we were building three new buildings, adding hundreds of products, computers many people and thousands of dollars in inventory.

I was helping them see small successes and continued getting small raises and even front money to buy a new mobile home at the beach that would be paid back over the first few years by way of additional, unobtrusive bonuses, and would become a summer home after that first year. I was still way behind where I was a year earlier, but felt appreciated and that I was being treated fairly, and with respect. I was asked to come back up north a year later and manage the new divisions and hire and manage the required employees as well as the outside sales force, which was growing rapidly as well.

He wanted me based north, but I told him I would settle in Dover, in the middle since I had to cover the whole state and because of June being employed south. Over the next two years, June commuted several months and switched jobs to Dover working for another medical outfit and I continued staffing the new buildings and positions while driving up and down the state. Financially, we were gaining on what we once had with June's help and steady increases and the promised bonuses on my part and moving in the right direction. We purchased our current home in Dover on two wooded acres and kept the beach home for a few years and then sold it.

June changed retail jobs several times always improving her situation landing in a inside sales position with my company, not working directly for me, but the manager of the Dover branch. I had six department managers working for me and continued as outside sales manager as well as the business continued to build on itself and soon was promoted to General Manager, but we were heading into another economical slowdown and things would begin to worsen, once again. June was last in, first out after more than a year in her position and moved again, to another retail position and continued to do well. We realized it was better for us also, because it is never too good of an idea working with a spouse, even if not working with him/her directly, because it sparked shop talk, not the kind of talk we needed.

June and I as a couple were doing ok. We supported each other, Shannon was in HS and Chris in JHS trying his hand in sports and learning fast. If you are monitoring me, I am still me, deeply as ever in love with June, but not able to visibly express it the way I know I could and should.

I want to note here, that some of these editorial expressions of self awareness on my part are not true representations of me at that time, as I was not as aware as I portray at the time of the writing, but am incorporating what I learned years later to try and explain what was happening. I have also, only recently discovered some of the problems that were occurring between us, by looking backwards.

Years later, when Shannon was younger, June and I were talking with her and she told us that I had changed while in Vietnam. Of course I jumped at her and said that she wasn't even a thought in our heads, before I shipped to Vietnam, how on earth would she know. She admitted that she had read letters she found while snooping around in closets as kids do. Letters, cards, even June's graduation board cap which had every visible inch covered by my writings with expressions of my love. I had given these to June while we were dating and she kept it with the letters from Vietnam. She compared the writings of then, to the actions and cards of now, and could tell that I gave her mom a lot more love and attention back then, since she had been old enough to watch us, and further felt that she and Chris had also been slighted by me.

Shannon was about 17 years old, but much older in her understanding of affection and emotion, when she told us that. I had neglected June for 19 years and did not have a clue as to how much and how bad it must have hurt her, and driven us apart to the point of divorce. The only way to show that was happening was to add my awareness which was definitely not easy, as this example was the first I was challenged with it from anyone other than June, and I obviously didn't hear her or didn't want to hear her all the time. I am listening and hearing her now and will continue to as long as I live.

My final job change began at the eleven year mark with the building material company. Things were getting rough as the economy was heading down again and my relationship had begun deteriorating a few years before that. Financially, the company was doing well, having more than tripled the sales in that time period, but I was having difficulties partly caused because of the husband/wife tandem as my superiors. I was often posed to agree with one over the other and back the other way again. I worked for him, but she owned the business so it was always a no win situation for me. Both were very nice people, but it was just an awkward situation for me to continue in. They also had three capable children and spouses that were now old enough to need jobs and others were moved in some instances to make room as well as new jobs created. There were other issues as well involving that old standby money. I had been promised a few years earlier that I would reach a prominent plateau, which was a milestone I was long in search of. I made great strides in the beginning and middle, however things started shifting around with the actual business and the results later on.

A couple years had passed since the original target date was issued and passed. We had several conversations, other factors of management issues and management styles began to change and I felt the need for a change. June had moved several times during that period also and jobs rallied and slumped, but she steadily worked on. I finally went to my boss and told him I thought I needed to leave, because I didn't feel like I could work for him anymore. I explained it to him completely, of course he disagreed because mostly it was about the way he handled some employees. I asked him to explain my situation to his wife and he said he would. Several more months passed with him avoiding me whenever possible until I cornered him one day and asked if he talked to his wife.

He hemmed and hawed and finally said yes, and she doesn't want you to leave. I looked at him and asked, AND? He shrugged and walked off. I started looking immediately, as secretly as possible.

After a while, I was contacted by, the son and part owner of a local, competitive business. He was a junior owner with his father senior, and three other siblings minor partners. The product mix was similar, but had some distinctive differences. I went through a series of meetings between the son and father, the only sibling involved other than financially, and a personnel consultant.

I was employed at the fourth session, with the blessing of the consultant, I believe sewing up the deal. We agreed that I would finish up the current year with my present employer and begin at the beginning of the year, because, the year end bonuses were presented as the Christmas bonus. They certainly understood as it was a sizable bonus for me and I wasn't going to leave it on the table as it was a result of the current years effort.

I ended up quitting at the end of the week of the bonus, two weeks before the end of the month, because my policy had always been, when someone wants to leave, it is best for all concerned to leave. No need to have an employee wanting to change or quit a job, stay around and explain to other employees and customers why he/she was leaving, especially a key manager. He wanted for me to stay, but his wife overruled him, I believe, and I left that day and promised to not go after his employees or customers. A promise I kept, but almost 20 employees and many customers followed me over the early years because they each asked me, I did not ask them.

We had to take a pay cut, standard operating procedure for them until you proved yourself, especially with the bonus unknown because it was both a calculated amount and included a performance factor as well. June was happy for me because I was beginning to bring a lot of angst home with me and that was unusual, but she was also concerned as we were starting over again with a good bit of uncertainties, Shannon was working and recently had her first son Kyle and Chris was beginning HS and sports with a great entry into football and wrestling from JHS.

Work was rough for the first year as it was an older company with a lot of people in positions they didn't deserve and hoping that I would disappear if they made it too tough for me. The son was my direct boss and I was hired as sales manager of all sales and store manager to start. The father was happy I was there to help and mentor his son but wanted the business to stay status quo, without many changes in personnel and products. My boss and the consultant agreed during the meeting my first morning, but as soon as the door closed, the other two scooted me into an adjacent office and said that they agreed with the father, but wanted me to start pressing the son when I saw opportunities and had ideas. I had almost walked when the father said that, because in my meetings with the other two, they stressed growth, that's why I wanted the job, to show what I could do and quickly, not to come and keep things as they were.

Time started flying as the first year closed and I began to act on everything I had observed during the year, as we had agreed. I started making changes and soon took over the operations part of the business also, and began adding and improving products and services, with the help and approval of my boss, and our combined and sure explanations to the father. This is when past employees and customers sought me out and I began accommodating them as business started booming, along with increases in the economy.

In addition to the remaining inherited employees, those that followed me and some great finds, we started to make headway with the newer products as well as the existing products. My pay started increasing at better than normal annual increases and June and I got involved as officers in both boosters clubs and never missed a game or match, a precondition of my employment, as I promised to give much more than 40 hours but would not miss an event. The sports and parental involvement were good for us, but might have disguised some aggravation on our part.

We had a great relationship with a lot of friends and were busier than ever before. We ran and worked many other boosters projects like a part time job, such as sports programs, team pictures, ad sales, shopping for tournaments and running the tournaments, concession stands, etc.

The rest of the decade rushed by, with my position increasing to General Manager and adding new branches in the middle and southern parts of the state. Shannon had her second son Kam, and started a good progressive career with a California company and the following year, Chris started at the U of Delaware following graduation. He did not want to pursue sports while in college as he felt burned out, didn't declare a major and didn't really enjoy it very much. Like Father like son, I guess, dropped out at the winter break and was shipping out to Parris Island for basic training and a five year enlistment in the Marine Corp, as a specialized aviation electronic technician.

I was steadily improving inside the company which had seen almost an six times growth in sales and four time growth in employees, all with a growing economy, great employees, vendors, products and customers, so I guess you know what's coming.

June began transitioning to part time retail sales jobs with a friend of hers in order to take a little time off, relax a little, thereby helping a slightly fractured hip heal while supporting herself with crutches. I was happy whatever she did as long as she was happy, and we worked on a lot of projects at home, like always as well as help replace the voids of the absence of the kids. Chris got married to Angelica just after his tour/cruise on a ship to the Kuwait area during the Iraq war added another eight months to his tour. She was from California and moved here to start their family following Chris' discharge and start of a career with our company, while she worked retail, in a push through job from her company in CA.

My job naturally slowed down with the big drop in home building, but not before I had been promoted to VP and been made a small financial partner, that yielded wonderful dividends. Incidentally, I blew past my previously unattained benchmark in several years and never glanced back. While that was happening, Chris and Angelica had their first daughter, Isela and June had retired for good so that she could watch Isela during the week until school began, which was curtailed by my getting sick, a few months following Shannon and her husband Johny's daughter Makenzie's birth.

I have had many of the problems of other Vietnam vets, but I feel I was able to deal with them better than a lot because June wouldn't let me drown in the rough times, even though I wasn't always very good company for her or our kids. A lot of those times are times I regret along with others I have mentioned. We didn't really know what a lot of those hard times were until years later and I've always shied away from blaming anything or anyone but myself. Once PTSD (Post Traumatic Stress Disorder) began being discussed openly as many of the Vietnam Era veterans were being diagnosed, did we start relating some of our situations and my complaints toward that possibility, but I never sought help. Many years and unexplained negative situations resulted from that unknown information, and damages went un-repaired for many, veterans, spouses and children, even grandchildren, as well as parents, siblings and grandparents.

I am eternally grateful to June and proud as a couple for fighting through all of the bad times, especially the separation we struggled with and came back from described earlier. I believe we were truly made to be together to take care of each other to the best of our abilities and further believe that we both did everything possible to that end, with the knowledge we had available. It wasn't always pretty or textbook, but we trusted in each other to keep it going.

June and I were alike in many ways, which has its good and bad points. I was looking for the right girl to spend the rest of my life with early on, probably because I felt that I needed a companion more than she felt that she did. Once we were together and things became serious enough to become engaged in August 1968, for about a year, I was drafted. We weren't going to get married yet because things started happening so fast. Drafted in June, 1969 her 19th birthday, physical on July 20, the first moon landing and Sissy's birthday, and shipped off to basic training in September. After three months of basic training I was assigned to the Infantry at graduation and right off to AIT (Advanced Infantry Training) for ten more weeks, destined to Vietnam after a two week leave.

Luck intervened, again, and toward the end of training I was interviewed and chosen for NCO (Non Commissioned Officer) school after AIT, specializing in Infantry Operations and Intelligence. Following a three day leave, three months of school, and three months of OJT (On the Job Training) at an Infantry Division in the states and thirty days leave before shipping to Vietnam. As AIT continued, I realized I had a three day leave coming my way during the Christmas break, followed by four more weeks of training. A slight opening, and marriage plans began to develop beginning that Christmas Eve and were finalized the day after Christmas. Wedding bells were going to chime the following month!

The above writing began approximately six months after I began psychiatric counseling following June's death in 2012, after my counselor and I had gotten on comfortable ground. All on me because I had to be one of the world's biggest skeptics in any type of counseling. I always felt that if I or my wife and I couldn't fix anything wrong with us, no one could, end of conversation. At the urging of my oncologist and some longtime friends, including Jeff who introduced me to June and lost his wife, my friend Shari in 2000 to cancer, I decided to give the VA clinic a try. Voila, my counselor had been trying from the beginning after discovering my recall for the past and, I guess my talking skills, suggested I try my hand at writing my experiences down, even offering a friend who was a court stenographer to assist. I kept shying away but as she was being so persuasive and nice to me, I decided to give it a try, sans the stenographer because of my shyness, and started picking away at writing these remembrances, to give my reading a little break. My counselor was never aware that I did anything but make notes about dreams and spiritual experiences that I had following June's passing, as we both experience spiritual events as do two other friends and I, and as June and I always did.

10/24/17

It has been approximately five years since I finished the previous notes session about some of my personal feelings following June's death on 8/8/12. I had evidently written them on June's personal computer and forgotten about doing it, my recent recall obviously not nearly as strong as my historical recall. Earlier this year I was looking for some of our old photos and ran across those notes and put them aside after reading them over and over.

I was in the middle of remodeling the master bathroom (June's) when June took the turn for the worst. I hadn't let her see anything except the floor tile and I let her pick out the colors by giving her curtains to choose from and knowing that she wanted a fairy garden theme as she loved and collected fairy figurines, books and pictures. I always liked to surprise her with everything possible, whenever possible, the more extreme, the better. I had just finished the heated floor tile, which I didn't even tell her about to surprise her, and was beginning to add all of the fixtures and cabinets when she had to go to Penn Cancer Hospital following her last collapse.

She never saw her bathroom and I just couldn't bring myself to work on it for years, because I was trying so hard to finish it so she could sit in the walk in tub and watch the hidden mirrored TV, or at worst, at least see it. At my counselor's urging again, I know, she is very good, I did finish it about two years later, after a short hospital stay.

I have been hospitalized three times since June's passing. New Years Eve 2012, early July 2014, and August 20, 2016. All three of those admissions involved me having hallucinations, running a slight fever associated with various maladies, and mostly, feeling deeply depressed about being without the woman I had loved so long and gone through so many ups and downs together as a team. I have also been prescribed morphine for my cancer related bone pain and neuropathy, since my diagnosis and chemo. It is important to note that I have been having VA psychiatric counseling as well as my therapy sessions, but my progress mostly rests with my counselor. My hospital stays ranged from four days to two weeks for the most recent stay which included a self-admittance to the VA Mental Hospital after an attempt to commit suicide.

Although that attempt came on the heels of the four year anniversary of June's passing, it was not due to the overwhelming feeling of remorse, but hallucinations and voices indicating, that was the way of being with June again. No need to go into the sordid details at this time, as that will be the final part of this book. However it is noteworthy that afterwards, realizing I was violating a nonverbal commitment to my family and friends to fight through all of the issues facing me, as well as to myself and June, I decided to do something about my situation. Not able to contact anyone because of my mental capacity and an inability to operate the phones and computer successfully, I very carefully drove myself to the local ER.

From the onset, I admitted fully what had happened and through daily meetings with a panel of doctors, nurses, specialists and group therapy sessions I was released from the very militaristic setting approximately ten days later. It was very similar to being back in the service where you had to make your bed, stand in line for everything, including vitals, teeth brushing, haircuts, meds, telephones and meals. Meetings throughout the day and evenings, shaving under supervision, etc. As a Draftee, needless to say, I hated it and vowed to never put myself or my family in that situation again. I haven't come close since, other than a rough adjustment period of a few weeks after coming home and almost driving my son loco as he unselfishly attempted to administer twice per day medications, in spite of having a two month old daughter, working full time and helping Angelica with the other two, a new dog Casper and karate and dance classes. I was a lousy patient, as we temporarily developed the child becoming the parent syndrome as Mom and I had two years earlier.

Once home and under a strict weekly follow up procedure with my VA medical and therapy team I began a very rigorous self evaluation and with doctors reluctant approval removed myself from most of my medications. No chemo, no pain medication, no mood regulating drugs. The only meds I was taking was for my blood pressure, and Acetaminophen for pain.

I have been in a better frame of mind and physical being since then and have managed to accomplish many things that went undone for four years. I tackled the overgrown gardens and yard work that I had let go because they were always projects that June and I enjoyed working on together. I finished the decks and stairs that I had started before I got sick. I went through the house again, attic, garage and outbuildings and reorganized (I still could not get rid of June's favorite clothes, coats/jackets and especially any shoes, which still occupy her side of the closets and always will as long as I'm here.) I got vehicles running and cleaned up. June's 51st surprise Birthday present a spa yellow pearl 2001 Honda S2000, still with just 6,700 miles, which she loved and we used for get away trips. And a 1973 red VW bug that I compulsively bought a few years after June passed because it was very similar to the brand new red Bug we had to buy her the day before I left for Vietnam, as hers died on the way back from our final day of leave at the beach. That was a huge relief at the time for me not to have to worry about her commuting to work and having her independence while I was away. I saw this one advertised on eBay, made an offer and picked it up a few days later with the help of my grandson Kyle driving my truck back from West Chester. All strictly on impulse of good memories and obviously a real weakness of mine and one I feed too often.

When it became a little too intense with the heat and humidity I moved up my "Fall" scheduled project of remodeling the kitchen/pantry/laundry room from subfloor up. I am in the clean up phase of that three month project at the present time. I feel relieved and proud that I have accomplished a lot by myself, with new subfloor, tile (floor and wall), ceilings, lighting, electric, plumbing, cabinets and countertops. The only thing I subbed out to contractor was the granite tops which I obviously can't do, although I had constructed our old laminate tops and backsplash.

I'm looking forward to continuing on other projects to keep myself occupied and typically begin purchasing products well ahead of actually beginning the work. We had bought the kitchen floor tile seven years ago in anticipation of that project beginning between my diagnosis and June's illness. Finally got to use them and stayed with the colors and design that we had originally intended.

I have frequent and needed meals and visits with family, friends and VA counselor which help keep me grounded. I read a lot to help keep my mind occupied. I have shifted somewhat my reading material but continue to keep my mind involved with the writings of the Vietnam war along with mysteries, thrillers, scientific and spiritual works. I also stay current on the treatment progress and statistical data with Multiple Myeloma and breast cancer.

My oncologist retired in the summer of 2016 and I had to return to the private sector for a year until the VA replaced him. I was told I was in remission at that time and asked to be removed from chemo, but continued the Zometa to help counter the bone loss of the Myeloma. Always in the front of my mind has been the original statements from my doctors that MM was not curable and would never stay in remission. Having returned to the VA oncology care this summer with a new doctor that I like, I have gone through routine testing and procedures. A recent MRI showed a problem area in my hip and required a PET scan which I had within three weeks. Those results showed a number of issues primarily with bones, but also some calcification on a lung, kidney and some blockage in heart and arteries, and diverticulosis. That dictated bone biopsies under the guidance of MRI which I had with mixed results, but nothing severe enough other than continued monitoring.

Some additional medical histories which tie in with my condition follow. I was diagnosed with Ischemic heart disease in 1991 after succumbing to pressure from my wife and mother following my brother Lee's early death (45) of a massive heart attack. That diagnosis was through my civilian physicians which I had at the time. I had intentionally stayed as far away as I could from the VA at that time because of the reputation it had throughout and immediately after the Vietnam Era.

In addition, June's father had passed away at the VA hospital after a bout of gout and toe amputation. The reason I bring this up is because Ischemic Heart disease is on the Agent Orange list of attributable diseases. To qualify for any benefits from that, you had to be diagnosed in the VA system. That was seventeen years before I was diagnosed with MM and my son notified me of the VA rights discussed in the earlier writing. I am not complaining because I am 100% covered as noted previously, but that could have been seventeen years of help prior to MM and possibly could have developed into an earlier diagnosis.

I wonder how many veterans are truly out there who are either unaware of these situations that drastically could effect their and their families lives, or are no longer with us that received no help at all. It is amazing to me how many vets are unaware of the dangers involved, just from my limited conversations with other vets during visits to the hospital. From that perspective I feel that I am again, a lucky individual and would love to find a way to have them all checked out.

I was viewed by friends and have always personally felt that I was "lucky". Mom said maybe because I weighed 7 lbs 11 ounces at birth or was born on 3/1/47, combinations of 7 &11, but not so lucky per my first fleecing while playing craps in the army. I have always been able to bounce back after small setbacks whether physical or mental, seemingly in the best place at the time, not necessarily the right place at the right time, but the best at a time I could make things work. And important for me in my condition, I have a very high threshold for pain. At the end of my Vietnam tour, my hooch and the one next to it were hit by rockets the day and time I was scheduled to take a dispatch Jeep to Division in order to process out and head back to the states. Instead of waiting for the jeep, I caught a flight with a helicopter pilot friend and left a few hours early. One of my friends was killed and several wounded in that incident. I also felt I had several other very fortunate situations for me, but unfortunate for others who suffered greatly, during my tour, as did most veterans.

Being chosen to go to NCO school out of AIT instead of directly to Vietnam was the luckiest for me because it gave June and I that window of opportunity to get married. We had decided to get married before I left for Vietnam so we could be together as husband and wife.

It was the worst snow storms in South Carolina in many years and graduation day from AIT. We were dismissed early and told to leave base before they closed the base to automobiles. I had to drive 900 miles to get to my own wedding the next day. I had promised to pick up my uncle who was going to our wedding and lived about fifty miles southwest of Ft. Jackson and had also promised two South Carolina friends to take them home as well as two others who lived in Delaware.

First we scrambled together our gear, all of it since we were traveling to new bases, drove through the gates and headed for my uncle's home. It took us twice as long as there was no traffic and much snow. We got to his home, loaded his bag and squeezed together because it was a small stick shift Rambler. The first drop off was south and then back north and east for the second. A few hours later we were finally on I95N and headed home, with a bit more room. We had heavy snow until the North Carolina, Virginia line, where it just disappeared but was following us north. We finally made it to my parents' house late Saturday morning after dropping the two local men at the closest ones' home.

June was off and came over so we could all go over Sundays plans and rehearse what little we had to rehearse. All of that done, June and I spent most of the rest of the day talking and laughing about finally getting married, but somewhere along the way I made her mad and she told me to take her to her Mom's home.

We got in the car and I begged her to forgive me for whatever I said and kept making it worse to the point she said she was not going to marry me and made me drop her off near her Mom's, so I wouldn't try to con her Mom to let me go in with her. I let her out and started driving around and around for a few hours thinking, until I finally drove back home and went to bed. The next morning I went out and bought her a nice card and flowers and sat down to write how very much I needed her and wanted her to be my wife, and again begging to be forgiven for making her mad at such the wrong time.

Hoping I had come up with the right words, since I obviously couldn't speak the right words, I took them to her home and knocked on the door, gave them to her Mom and waited in the cold car. A short while later she came out and we made up. All was well, but I was still scared, until she presented a card to me, it read, and I still have it, "My Dearest Lover Bub, You would have to throw me off a cliff to keep me from marrying you! Your June, Forever".

We had a beautiful, quaint, small wedding that was, in both our minds better than any other we ever attended. Her brother gave her away and they came down the stairs as my Dad played the Wedding March on the organ, then stood with me as he was my best man also. My mother and both grandmothers were there with my brother, his wife and daughter. June's mother, aunt and two cousins.

My uncle and a cousin with his fianc . Four of June's friends from work including her bridesmaid, several family friends, one doing the photography, and the Reverend and his wife. After a drink of champagne, a bite of cake, off we went into the snow again, next stop Atlantic City, NJ, but casinos were almost ten years in the future, and the famous boardwalk and steel pier was not open. It was the only place we thought of, because it was the nearest beach that was open at all and the beach is where we spent our time together whenever possible. We had a quiet day and half and headed back home in a mild snow storm.

Upon the completion of my NCO school of three months, my parents and June flew the Cessna to Ft. Benning and joined me after my graduation and promotion to Sgt E-5, 11F40, Infantry Operations and Intelligence. We then flew back home, got in Dad's Rambler and she and I drove back to Columbus, GA where we rented a quaint small two bedroom mobile home which was our first time alone, other than our two day honeymoon. We were able to find each other as husband and wife in total solitude, except for my extended duty hours and the kitten which apparently came with the home. All very lucky indeed. We drove to Panama City, Florida almost every weekend I wasn't on duty because we both loved the beach so much and had spent as much time as possible at the Delaware/Maryland beaches while dating.

It was during my OJT that I really started to see some of the petty antics that were used in the service. I was assigned to a unit that was staging returnees from Vietnam and utilizing us as workers around base as well as burial details for returning local KIA's. I made two friends quickly who had just returned from Vietnam and the Cambodia incursion who were brothers who served in the same unit at the same time, one being Sgt E-5, the other and two year younger Spec 4. As we began working together in the orderly room and ceremonial burial details, they began telling me their stories of what things were like over there and they painted a tough somber picture which definitely heightened my concern. They were also going over the secrecy and intrigue of their operation and were very descriptive and suggestive to me about their daily routines. As we continued to move through the details and daily clerical work we were assigned, a new major was introduced and wanted to start rigorous PT and running conditioning after work for these men just in from Vietnam.

I had just finished the massive running and PT in NCO school and wanted no part of it because that took my time from being with June. Everyone who could, avoided the exercise details and he had poor turnout, so he began walking around just before we finished our work details and corralling all that he could. I got caught in some, and of course hated the running in June, and July weather in southern Georgia. I began slipping away, with many, many others as often as possible. That continued for a good while, until he began coming into the orderly room talking to the Captain and Lieutenant who I worked for, complaining that I wasn't participating like I should.

They liked me because I was a better typist than any permanent people they had and took care of the detailed and difficult tasks, so they started loading me up until he came through saying that the work was more important. At some point, the major realized that I was next stop Vietnam where the others were returning from, and it hit the fan. He started running me down, verbally challenging me personally that I wasn't tough enough to make it over there and I would surely not be able to handle it and probably not make it back home.

He even enlisted the brothers to engage me and pile on with their war stories and enforce the fact that I wouldn't make it if I weren't in tip top shape. It actually became somewhat comical, as I had the attitude of, what are you going to do to me, send me to Vietnam, because I've already got my order date? I told him that I had just gotten married and I was intent on spending as much time with my wife as I could just in case I didn't come back. He even followed me to my car on occasion basically calling me a wuss, while I drove the little rambler off. He never tried to order me, and I would give him a win occasionally but sneak out of the run when we got near the parking lot.

What did I care, I was never going to see any of these people again, and everyone else was doing the same thing, but they were already vets of the war and I wasn't, so he chose me to pick on.

The games continued, and they had me start processing through all of the medical and dental checkpoints about three weeks early, so I could go to one station per day at the end of the day and avoid the runs. He would see me walking with a folder and remind me of the run, and I would say that I was processing that day. I even started crossing the street when I saw him so as not be required to salute him and that made him livid. I skated as much as possible, gave and took, and started building up my gripes about the green machine. The brothers were having a ball helping me and informing me about how the statistics were obtained and accumulated, and bragged even at this low level, using their units statistics and cache results as examples. I was soon to start seeing what they were talking about first hand, and saw also how the senior people would treat the newer people, and I wasn't even there yet. Boy was I in for some surprises about how shit rolls down hill in Vietnam, but would be pleasantly surprised as well because some of the friends I made.

A required thirty day leave followed. That would put me in the position of DEROS (Date Return from Overseas Service) at the end of my one year tour. The Army did not want to bring back draftees to the States and have them mix with domestic enlisted soldiers because of their negative feelings about the war or to pass on subpar disciplinary attitudes and tendencies to new soldiers with only months of obligation remaining, as I had been doing without even being there yet. DEROS was the preferred way of accomplishing this.

At the end of my OJT, I collected my travel orders for Vietnam and back to Delaware we headed, towing a trailer with our meager belongings to my favorite Spartanburg, South Carolina, grandmother where we wanted to visit Lee, working in a factory as he and Leslie had just separated for several months to work out some problems. Lee picked Spartanburg because my grandmother lived there and he rented a small room near by. I went to the factory, where I found his motorcycle and left a note on his seat that we were in town and I was headed to Vietnam in 30 days and would love to see him. He did come over the next morning and wished me good luck, smacked June and my Grandmother on their butts, and off we went, my favorite Grandmother in the back seat of my Father's old Rambler, my beautiful wife beside me.

That month flew by, visiting family and friends saying goodbye and ended with a week at the beach and the dying VW bug. The following day June and I headed back to my friend and left with the new 1972 red bug, and a few hours later my Dad and I decided it best that we go to the airport alone. Probably easier on all but June and I. My new wife, Mother, both Grandmothers, two year old niece Shelly, Leslie and trusty Puppy Dawn were lined up on the sidewalk in front of the house as I went down the line and back to June for the last hugs and kisses. No dry eyes, especially mine. It was an almost silent drive to the Philadelphia airport with my Dad driving, where I was scheduled to fly to Ft. Lewis, WA via Chicago.

I had decided to wear civilian clothes and put my khaki uniform in a bag and change in a rest room in Seattle before getting on the bus to Ft. Lewis. I didn't have to wear my uniform on the flight because I didn't fly via service member standby, as my Dad had made reduced fare reservations through his airline connections. My hair had grown a bit in that month of leave, which aided a little to the disguise to avoid any interactions with other travelers who might have things to say about the war, which was very common. It was almost always encountered and we were told to bite our tongues and remember who we were. We usually did. I always did. I had many other things on my mind.

My Dad a commercial pilot and very familiar with most airports, especially Philadelphia, amazingly positioned himself in strategic terminal windows so that every time I had a view of the terminal during my taxi out, I would see him. He had white bucks on and one foot up on the sill of the window at every siting, like he was a wandering statue. I will never forget that sight. He also flew many DC 8 plane loads of soldiers to Vietnam before and after my trip, and even increased those trips during my tour hoping for a chance for us to see each other. That opportunity never presented itself, however he was able to carry a few "care packages" to Vietnam and bypass that first giant step.

I had a layover in Chicago and spent the entire time on the observation deck. A hot, humid late September day, although not comparable to the morning I disembarked in Cam Rahn Bay, Vietnam a few days later in the unforgettable, odorous steam bath I would always remember. I had a love affair with my first live sighting of the new Boeing 747's that were in and out of the traffic patterns at the Chicago O'Hare airport. They seemed suspended in air as they floated like bumble bees onto the runway and powered up, seemingly incredibly vertical in their takeoff ascent. Understanding the science of flight, having earned my commercial pilots license a few years earlier, I was still amazed at their ability to simply fly, and wanted to fly in one in the worst way. Ironically, I did on my return flight from Vietnam, via Ft. Lewis and Chicago back to Philadelphia.

There were about seven of us in brand new summer greens with our new colorful ribbons and braids loaded alone in first class, kept apart from the rest of the passengers in a flight leaving Washington in the wee hours of the morning. We assumed it was to avoid any disturbances with the other terminal passengers. We had all received angry looks and some comments in the sparsely attended Ft. Lewis terminal after midnight. Remember, this was the tail end of the war and servicemen and women were not usually respected, but attempts at humiliation were all too often. We didn't care because we had the 'stewardesses' to ourselves and they and the rest of the crew treated us like kings serving us free drinks and snacks while the curtains were pulled between cabins. More about the beginning of this trip later.

June continued to work and lived with my parents while I was in Vietnam. We rented an apartment within a week after my return and had a blast shopping for our first pieces of furniture. We took my favorite Grandmother with us and used her sage advice of not being cheap with our mattress set as we wouldn't get a new one for many years. We got an expensive Queen set which lasted us until we moved into our current home and replaced it with another expensive king, Grandmothers' advice everlasting.

I started taking classes at the U of D and got a night shift job on the Chrysler assembly line right away. We had her one year old VW bug but I needed transportation for work and school so I bought a small Honda motorcycle for commuting. After one winter of driving in snow and rain, we got rid of the cycle and bought another used bug from family friends. Those were our cars from 1972 until we traded her bug in1976 for a Granada and mine in1978 for a

Pinto. At that final trade, my VW had a plywood rear floor supporting the battery underneath the seat, as mine had recently fallen through to the road. The plywood worked just fine and that was the first thing I checked on the one I purchased a few years back. No plywood, no rust.

To finish up my life with the early years, I'll start with my Dad learning how to fly as an early teenager, not far off the coast in South Carolina. Dad began flying at the ripe old age of 14 in Walterboro, the home of the Tuskegee Airmen, the first Negro pilot training group in the Army Air Corp. He was not connected to that unit at all as it was much earlier, but began flying as a utility pilot towing banners over Charleston beaches and crop dusting locally, primarily. He joined the Army Air Corp after almost a decade of flying and flew many different transports throughout the Europe and Africa theaters as a Captain, came back to the states and landed in Nashville, Tennessee where he met and married my Mom, where she and her two sisters were working for the government in the war effort as secretary, typists.

Mom and Dad shortly moved to Florida, where my brother Lee was born in Miami, on May 16, 1945, toward the end of the war and shortly the new family moved back to the Nashville area when I was born in Murfreesboro, Tennessee, on March 1, 1947, where my Dad finished his enlistment. After the war he began training Air Force pilots, as a civilian instructor, in North American T6's Texans trainer aircraft, in Moultrie, Georgia where we had relocated and my brother and I started grade school. While in Georgia, President Eisenhower would fly into Spence Air Base, when he played golf in Augusta, home of the Masters Golf Championship. His pilot was a good friend of my Dad's and they flew together during the war. On one trip Colonel Draper let us tour Airforce One, rather the "Columbine", as the president named the first official plane prior to being designated as Airforce One, the radio call sign of the airplane flying the President at the time. We had a family picture with the colonel in front of the Columbine and took a tour.

In the middle 1950's Dad took a job with Capitol Airways, a cargo carrier, as operations manager and pilot and we moved up north to Delaware, in 1955. Capitol grew quickly from cargo to passenger carrier and he flew the beautiful and streamlined tri tail Lockheed L-1049 Super Constellation four propeller passenger airliners. He continued as operations manager and added Chief Pilot to his credentials around the time I was beginning junior high school and by the time I started high school, the company included a fleet of Douglas DC8 Stretch jet airliners. After a year wrangling both jobs, he left the operations job, as his love of flying the new jets took precedence, and he had his choice on the bid list of flying his favorite charter flights all over the world. He continued his glamorous, albeit lonely career and retired at age sixty in 1979, an FAA regulation which has since been raised to sixty-five.

I followed Lee throughout our school years doing my best to live up to his athletic achievements in football, wrestling and throwing the javelin in track. He set a great example for me, as a big brother, as well as many targets to shoot at in the athletic arena. We both had very successful junior high and high school careers and got to play one season together in three high school sports and one season of college football together, on opposite sides of the ball, me at center and Lee at middle linebacker. Lee went on and played four years as I retired as a sophomore with injuries, as mentioned earlier. Both parents were avid fans, but Mom was the full time supporter as Dad was traveling during many events, but always sent a telegram to the team to spur on a victory, while Mom was a spectacle in her own right, as her enthusiasm and spirit, more than made up for him when absent.

My brother Lee continued through college and got married in 1967 to his wife Leslie, while midway through school and they welcomed their only child, daughter Michelle a year and half later. Lee also started his pilot training, but stopped shortly before his final testing as he determined it wasn't for him. He had a very successful career as a VP, managing plants in the paper industry, but died at a young 45, on Mothers' Day 1991 upon leaving my house for the ER, during a major heart attack.

Leslie later remarried and continued her career. It was very difficult time for me, having lost my favorite grandmother a few years earlier, and not getting over either one very easily, especially not in a day, as I had once predicted. Many memories flooded my mind and pushed me into a depression that made me wonder what more I could have done to show them both that I loved them, like I really did.

Lee had always been mad at himself as the older brother for not going to Vietnam instead of me, but he was married and had a child. June and I were not married at the time and did not have a child.

AMBUSH

BOOK II: VIETNAM

Having given a mini version of my life history, a condensed auto biography of sorts, I have attempted to divulge some of my personality, feelings, and ideals about my life and life in general. This insight, along with adding some likely controversial subjects and statements about war, values and history is my goal in the remaining pages of this writing, in addition to filling in some missing pieces to my personal history. I hope to integrate these views with more of my life experiences, but not in the very detailed nature of writing, as if writing an historical accounting of the life of any soldier, including myself, in the Vietnam war.

June, my wife of forty two and two third years, passed away on 8/8/12, when I was sixty five years old. I had retired three years earlier after being diagnosed with non-curable Multiple Myeloma cancer, attributed to Agent Orange exposure. My reading habits up to this point in my life were best described as sporadic, reading several books per year, mostly novels about the war. June was the reader in our family and traded paperbacks regularly with family members, co-workers and friends until the E-book, followed by Kindle came along. She was usually curled up in bed reading, while I was channel surfing before falling to sleep.

I began reading as a way to fight off boredom and primarily to keep my mind occupied and distanced of the loss of my soul mate, in addition to being dramatically slowed down physically by my reactions to chemo and the associated maladies.

Many books have been written by Vietnam veterans from all services, units, ranks, etc., about their own experiences, and I have read between 250 and 300. This represents approximately 60% of books I have read in the five and half years since my wife passed away. The majority of those have been consumed during condensed periods of time, primarily winter, when I feel the most need to find something to keep my mind occupied.

Most of the books I enjoy greatly, all genres and my list also contains murder mysteries, thrillers, intrigue, spiritual, and historical, both novels and factual accountings, and range from a few hundred pages to one thousand plus. I usually stay with the book until I finish, finding time to eat, sleep and take care of necessary tasks and chores. My goal is to finish without too many interruptions, as I really do get into the book and have a strong desire to complete the story with a feeling of satisfaction and continuity. At times, I finish one book and buy another immediately on my Kindle, or on line if there is a new best seller I want to read, especially when I am on one of those binges I tend to force on myself.

Recently, I tried reading four books at the same time, finding good transition places in one and moving on to the others. These books were all the same genre, but very different authors, so it was quite difficult picking them back up and compartmentalizing to separate them completely.

This came about as a suggestion of another reader and friend of mine, as she suggested the method and subject books. I have to admit that I did not finish any of the books, but did get a very good understanding of each to be able to make comparisons and discuss with my friend.

I had reasons that I abandoned all four books and each one was a little different than the next. Ironically, my friend's journey was much the same. Of the other books during this time frame, I have less than a dozen not completed, mostly because of the quality of the writing or the content. I usually get interested very quickly and want to finish the story and when I do abandon a book, it is usually early on in the reading, so not much time is lost. Interestingly, my tendency to do the same thing with movies or television shows.

I'm writing this story for several reasons, most of the books I have encountered involving Vietnam veterans are those mentioned earlier, war stories. Most very good accurate accountings of what it was like to be a Soldier, Marine, Sailor, Airman, Coastguardsman, pilot, sniper, doctor, nurse, medic, reporter, or even an enemy soldier. All very interesting in all rights and informative from the perspective of someone who spent their time in country. Blending different perspectives from all sources provides a more complete picture of what life was like in country to me, for those individuals, to hopefully develop a feeling of composite experiences myself.

I would like readers to have an increased feeling of what things were like for returnees from Vietnam in relation to more than just what happened over there. I will try to describe some of the things I was experiencing and feeling as relates to my historical life in general, before shipping out and after my return. I can't speak for any other veterans, nor reflect an accurate depiction of most and certainly, not all.

No two people are the same as we all know, and every dramatic little thing we encounter in our life can change direction of the course we were headed on. Like tacking in the wind and water currents in a boat, or correcting a flight path in an airplane with the winds aloft reports obtained from weather stations. A constant correction of course is required to achieve your desired destination, but on slightly different courses, and in the case of our life, we don't always know the exact destination, do we? And if you can look back at yourself at age 18-23, or are that age or younger, try to reclaim your goals at the time, and your direction and destination. Were you absolutely sure, are you sure, or will you be sure when you reach that age? I think the overriding answer is no, I don't think it is likely.

I will not apologize for any harsh words used to convey my views and descriptions of the soldiers from the Vietnam era because that would be misrepresentative and void of the realities of the times, but I will not exaggerate it either. I do apologize for using negative connotation slang words like gook and slant eyes, but for authenticity of the times and mindset.

I often explain to friends and family that the average GI inserted a curse word after every few words and sometimes every other word, and that is true as my experiences go.

It was just the way of life and portrayed a very harsh opinion of everything occurring on a daily basis, which was carried back with you when you came home for a period of time, depending on the individual and their self control. I'm quite certain that hard language is used in wars now, just as it was used in wars before and will be in those to come, very similar to athletes in tough contests and in locker rooms, or in angry arguments, only intensified dramatically. Frustration was the rule and a result of fear, loneliness, depression, uncertainty, lack of hope, and sheer anger directed in almost every direction at any time. Fear of the unknown being the constant, common denominator in most activities as in discussions.

I remember fearing most anything that was new and unknown to me the entire tour, in the field, in transit, in base camps, and fire bases. I personally tried to never "take a chance" trying anything new or unknown to me, as others would do. No touching anything that I couldn't 100% identify, no extraneous visits to the local villes for a "steam and cream" (a hot bath, massage, or more), a shopping or sightseeing trip into a city such as Hue, nor trips away from my immediate unit location other than absolutely necessary.

I didn't even go to the mess hall tent more than a handful of times while in the basecamp or fire bases, and not just because I hated the food and bug juice (watered down kool aid) as I usually ate C rations, stashed PX canned food stuffs, and those lovely care packages from home. Luckily, toward the end of my tour we began to obtain the newer LRRP (Long Range Reconnaissance Patrol) meals, now called MRE's (Meals Ready to Eat). And most important on my list of do nots, no drugs at all including marijuana. Most people smile in disbelief when I tell them I was in college four years in the late sixties and spent a tour in Vietnam and never even tried marijuana, but it is still true at age seventy-one.

I'm sure most newly returned veterans from any war, experienced a hackneyed phrase, such as "please pass the fucking potatoes Mom", or "what the fuck are you looking at asshole?", and so on. It was a challenge to negate a habitual routine like that which was the means of letting frustration and relief come out during your daily communications with buddies. I was lucky enough to slip only a few times my first few days home, with a gasp and stern look from my mother, at the dinner table, but smiles from my wife, brother, father, and grandmother.

I think the worst my Mom heard from my mouth prior to that was, " you shit ass", when I was five or six and extremely pissed at my brother. To my recollection, I had just recently heard that expression fired in anger from my father a few days earlier, and it seemed to stick and fit my needs at the time. I can still visibly remember standing in a field with my brother and friends after playing ball just as my brother had stopped the play because he didn't like the way it was going. I was yelling as loudly as possible, just what I thought of him as I saw my mother approaching in her car, seemingly in slow motion, windows wide open as there was no air condition back in the 40's and 50's, and looking my way.

Immediately, I knew I was in deep shit because of the look on her face and the smile on my brother's, chipped tooth and all. I received a long, strong tongue lashing on the ride home, my brother reveling at my discomfort, and I truly had my mouth washed out with soap for the first and only time, when we arrived at home. I'm not sure what brand! My brother often heard that and worse from me, and I from him, as he was always getting under my skin and creating bodily harm to me, as siblings do, but my parents were mostly always out of earshot. I still have scars on my head and face from some of the encounters with my big brother Lee, all naturally undeserved, being the younger, more calm, and non trouble making type, while he was the big bully brother type. Just kidding, we did have our issues, but he set goals for me in life and in sports by leading me by example and showing me how to compete with pride, and looked after me, as my big brother protector. I truly miss him now.

I grew up shy southern boy with a very quiet disposition and the grandson of a Baptist minister. That grandfather died during my first year, but I was raised in a religious atmosphere and taught the proper military and southern manners of always saying "yes sir, no sir, and yes ma'am, no ma'am", etc.

One afternoon in sixth grade, having moved to a new, northern Delaware town and changing school in the middle of the school year, I answered a science teacher by saying "yes sir" and he jumped all over me and told me to not call him sir. I was very upset and confused and ran home after school and told Mom what had happened. She consoled me, advised me that I was to always continue as I was taught and she would come to school the next day and straighten it out. She did come to school with me the next morning, explained to the principal what had taken place, and a few minutes later Mr. Z was standing in the office. After introductions, the three of us listened to my Mom expressing her contempt for him for degrading me in front of my classmates, simply for having manners, as taught, delivered with a Southern Belle's drawl and indignant conviction. Mr. Z never even gave me a sideways look after that day. Mothers, especially Southern ones, are very protective, and proper.

During wartime, cursing with enthusiasm was the way of communicating up, down and across the chain of command and could even become more vulgar when screaming at the enemy. Usually those exchanges occurred during firefights and nighttime encounters from perimeter to concealment in the jungle. Those shouting matches usually involved an unseen, or sparsely seen foe and involved the internationally popular comments about one's gook, or slant eyed mothers, following threats of "Fuck You GI, you die tonight", or "me croc-a-dao you GI" (kill you) occasionally accompanied by the shrill, falsetto cry of "faaa-cu" as a local gecko lizard enlightened the conversation with its mating call.

Those lizards, named by GI's as "fuck you lizards" were ever present at night and a scary introduction for FNG's (Fucking New Guy) thinking the enemy had found his location. The enemy's English vocabulary was very limited, but they could almost match our conversations of "go fuck yourself dumbass", "fuck you GI, you fucking boocoo dinky dau (very crazy)", or other soothing comments. Their sentences in English weren't very long or sweet, and were spoken from youngest to oldest, when necessary to communicate.

Other instances could be encountered during searches, road side purchases, or just passing by a village on foot on in a vehicle. A very common sight was a young male pimping his mother or sister, while making a circle of thumb and forefinger in one hand and pushing the middle finger of the other hand through it, with the sales pitch of "hey GI, sucky-fucky, two bucky my sister/mother". Or "you fucking number ten GI", the worst rank on 1 to 10, scale for flipping them the bird or yelling at them, ranging to "10 thou" if really bad, and " you number one GI" for tossing them a can of C rations, cigarette, candy bar, or other desirable, or souveniring it to them.

These are things that young eighteen year old GI's heard within their first few days in country to their last, as it was usually similarly, the extent of the Vietnamese' English conversation. In addition, kids would jump up on trucks trying to rip your watch off of your wrist while you were pointing an M16 right in their face, no fear at all. Kids of all ages, from just learning to walk and talk to just young enough not to be drafted into the South Vietnamese Army, or taken by the insurgents to fight the Americans, running beside your vehicles. Younger girls carrying sibling infants on their hips, begging for food, candy, gum, cigarettes and money. Old Mama sans with black teeth to toothless with black gums, from chewing mouth numbing black betel nuts, squatting where they stood to relieve themselves, young girls and boys trying to sell ice cold cokes for a buck. Lacking are middle aged women who are primarily working the fields or walking along the road carrying two loaded baskets or buckets on either end of a long pole or yoke over one or both shoulders and motoring down the dusty shoulder.

The older villagers usually squatted in the common oriental way, butt almost on their heels, and just watched you go by, and more importantly, and missing, are the 13 to 40 year old males, because of serving in the military of either side. Any closeup photograph of any of these subjects could have been the cover photo of a National Geographic Magazine. They truly displayed the face of the citizenry and refugees of a third world country conflicted in war and avoiding on a round the clock basis, becoming a collateral damage statistic later tallied as another historical result of war. We remember all too well, or have seen, those of a prisoner being shot in the head at point blank range, the hoards of refugees fleeing harm, and the little naked girl, burnt severely and running toward help, in pain and in shock, not even crying.

The sights and sounds were surreal and one of the instant impressions you would smack you between the eyes and remember your entire life. I had an immediate pity for what was happening to these poor civilians that never went away, but increased the more I was exposed to it. Riding through an ancient village of shacks of straw and bamboo, ammo crates, sticks and mud, sometimes sided with flattened American steel beer cans of all brands or derequisitioned PSP (Perforated Steel Plates), used for bunkers and field runway construction.

No toilets, no water, crude poverty, flanked by American logos of Coca Cola, Esso, Texaco, Shell, etc., on signs and buildings everywhere you look as you approached a populated area. Bicycles and Honda mopeds, water buffalo carts the primary transportation mode other than feet and bicycles, military vehicles and busses stacked to and high onto the roof with people, chickens, pigs, baskets of food, and personal belongings. As you entered a modern city, things would begin to look more civilized except for the obvious signs of war and the vast destruction of blown up buildings and bullet holes, Tet 1968 just two and half years earlier than my tour.

Most noticeable to me were the teenage university school girls, while driving through Hue, walking and riding bikes, dressed in traditional pajama sets, usually black or white, with colorful ao dai's, long, hi collar jacket like cover, usually brightly colored or white also. Their long, straight black hair streaming behind them, they were quite beautiful and seemed out of place among the refugees, war vehicles and destruction, as life tried to ignore the confusion. Anywhere you looked, there were paradoxes of old and new, and beautiful and dirty and purely obscene. Crumbling buildings surrounded by beautiful palm trees. Beautiful waterways jammed with sampans, rising above them, the rubble of ranks of destroyed buildings.

Horizons full of endless green and straw colored rice patties and reddish brown dikes, backed by dark green, purple hazed jungled mountains and on the other side of the road acres of emerald green, water filled bomb craters, jumbled together like craters on the moon except for color, backed by the beautiful blue and green of the South China

Sea. It was a beautiful country then, if you could extract the views of a savage and very destructive war, comparable to any Pacific Island paradise in weather, scenery and mystique, only too heavy on the mystique at that time in my life.

The heat and humidity has been chronicled in the majority of the books I have read, and movies watched, mostly as a first impression upon stepping from the freedom bird and onto the portable stairs upon arriving from civilization to the tropical war zone. For me, it was equally, extremely impressionable and made more retainable by the very unique and pungent assault on the olfactory and visual senses. The heat and humidity was unmatched to me, maybe because of being cooped up for 24 hours in an airplane, as you could actually see and smell the stale moisture in the air and outhouse like odors. The smell was a combination of hot, wet earth, with excrement added for effect, and the ever present mix of burning kerosene or jet fuel. Visual was the purple/gray haze in the air and the mirage like mirrored heat waves rising from the runways, the constant roar of jet engines and sounds of helicopters completed the sensual assault.

Many other memorable smells attacked you throughout your tour including nuoc mam sauce (pungent hot sauce for eating raw fish) and fish heads the local delicacy, the stench of the dead, the smell of rotten flesh from yourself and your buddies' rotted feet and body often unwashed for weeks on end, and most renowned, napalm and burning flesh (crispy critters the GI slang), and burning shit.

I was lucky enough to be put in charge of a shit burning detail during my first day of SERTS (Screaming Eagles Replacement Retraining School) classes, immediately upon reporting in to my unit, 101st Airborne/Airmobile Division. Most Divisions had a short training cycle for new soldiers to acclimatize, recondition, obtain local knowledge and zero your weapons, among many other training stations and reminders of all of the things to avoid, and your first turns on perimeter guard duty at night. At SERTS, we also did rappelling from a helicopter skid on a 40' tower and simulated a combat assault several klicks (1000 meters) west toward the mountains and infamous A Shau Valley, and the basic refresher courses of all of the do's and do not's while enjoying your one year tour, most noteworthy and memorable, the sapper demonstration in the mud and concertina wire by the repatriated NVA soldier, who made you realize how impossible a task it was to impede him.

Myself and three privates, wearing the new jungle fatigues, boots, and soft cap issued several days earlier before leaving Ft. Lewis, WA, were given a guide and escorted via truck to a portion of the many latrines throughout the large brigade combat base, Camp Evans. We worked into the night pulling half 55 gallon steel drums from each hole in single, to six hole latrines and dragging them with metal hooks, similar to bailing hooks with long handles, to the burning area near by, unavoidably splashing the contents all over ourselves.

The required use of daily malaria tablets issued a few days earlier with the primary doses on Sunday helped to create a very liquid and nasty slurry for the containers. The half cans were combined into one or two cans for burning, with two GI's gently lifting by the sides and pouring as delicately as possible. The empties replaced in the latrine slots with additional empty ones, while one of us added a recipe mix of kerosene and gasoline and stirred with a large wooden stick until the slurry was burning fully, while trying to stay upwind dodging the ever shifting, toxic smoke, usually to little or no avail. These steps repeated throughout the day.

It was advised to rap on the latrine and announce the procedure so that you didn't catch a sergeant or worse, an officer in mid bowel movement, pulling the can out from under him. If you did that, the proverbial shit would most definitely hit the fan, with you in front of the fan.

Yes, usually officers and some very senior NCO's had their own dedicated latrines, somewhat more elaborately constructed, which often got infiltrated in the early morning hours by enlisted men wanting a more sanitary and private experience. Oh, another piece of useful information; do not piss in the cans because they fill up too soon and add to the slopping for the unfortunate FNG "shit burning" crews, rather use the many four inch white tubes sticking out of the ground near all populated buildings, the piss tubes. Statistics show that approximately 90% of the GI's were diagnosed with severe diarrhea while in Country.

The following morning all newcomers, newbies, green peas, cherries, FNG's had to go to supply and turn in four of the five sets of new jungle fatigues, one of the two pairs of boots and one hat. We were all unknowingly used as part of the supply chain into the unit, having humped with us from Ft. Lewis, those extra clothing items, thinking they were ours for the duration. I requested and was begrudgingly allowed to exchange the uniforms, boots and hats my crew and I were still wearing, having slept in them that night, for new ones we carried in, to at least avoid the stink. It would not have been offered had I not asked.

The big rub with the procedure was that supply kept all the new fatigues for the people in the rear, REMF's (Rear Echelon Mother Fucker), or black market, and did not rotate the new in with the weekly resupply of laundered war torn fatigues supplied to the fighting units. The laundered, extremely worn fatigues were part of the weekly, or when possible, helicopter resupply to those out in the field and dumped in a big pile from the logistics helicopters. The soldiers had to sort through and choose from mis-matched and mis-sized uniforms, along with C rations, water, and ammunition. The saving grace of those resupply operations was mail call, if you were lucky enough to receive one or more letters, or the jackpot for you and your buddies, a care package from loved ones.

GI authors provide enormous reality from the in country point of view, dependent on their job MOS (Military Occupational Specialty) code, location, unit, season and time in country, etc. I soak all of that up in order to try to understand the various situations encountered by all of the authors I have read. What people experienced varied wildly as those categories mix and change. They change further by rank, gender, age, skin color and even religion. I believe that is what makes it so interesting to me and creates my thirst of learning by comparing these to my experiences, which helps to explain to people who asked over the last forty-seven years, THE question, "What was it like over there?" There just can't be a singular, uniform response to that question, as it surely has to be "in the eyes of the beholder", further developed by that person's personality, experiences and perceptions of life, before and after his/her tour, which is then usually tailored to those asking the question.

I usually try to take a more subdued approach to answering that question with generalities, mixing what I consider the common expected view, with my own experiences complying or competing with those perceived views. I often counter, what I consider to be the harsh impression depicted via the media and perceptions of the time, which points out more of my personality, because of being skeptical or not all believing as some want us to be.

Many of the facts reported back then were later proven to be false or misleading in order to prove points that were being made. That impression seemed to change significantly as time and casualties wore on, until it became a source of confrontation for many, which greatly impacted the impressions of civilians and soldiers alike. Not that I've been asked that question very often, which therein possibly lies one of the roots to the problems associated with Vietnam era veterans, that very few people actually wanted to know what it was like, they just didn't care and especially would not ask to be told or possibly were afraid to be told, many families included, and as a result, the damaging memories were held inside.

For me, that question was first asked by an Army PFC in the Seattle Airport around 1:00 AM on a hot summer morning, early June, 1971. I had returned from Vietnam the day before, received my honorary and complimentary steak dinner with all the trimmings, and began the steady grind of processing out of the war and the U.S. Army for good, along with my final cash payout which included my last monthly hazardous duty stipend of approximately $85.00.

I was ETSing (Expiration of Term of Service) and receiving my DD-214 (Department of Defense Certificate of Release or Discharge from Active Service) separation papers. I had three months remaining on my two year draft enlistment, but had received a three month drop to return home and go back to college and further my higher education as part of President Nixon's troop reductions, and Vietnamization program, with the aide of the GI bill.

The process was similar to the in processing the previous year, when leaving for Vietnam. However this time, I was one step away from going home to my beautiful wife of eighteen months, instead of leaving her. The primary procedural differences were much less hassle, a shorter process, a thorough drug test and physical, more shots, one new uniform to wear home, adorned with the colorful and useless medals and awards you were accorded.

And finally, for those that were lucky enough to ETS, possibly the last salute you would be required to give an officer. Those who were continuing their enlistment were going home on leave and would be issuing many more salutes and continuing the grind in the big green machine. The comparable main reward for all, was that we were back in the WORLD, which is what the USA was constantly referred to while in country, the home of the giant PX (Post Exchange)!

I was dressed in my brand new summer greens uniform, altered to fit my new lean body, which was destined to hang in my Mom's closet in less than 24 hours, for 40 years, adorned with my SGT stripes, 101st Airborne Screaming Eagle patch and three rows of medals, later removed and stuck in a box and stowed away with all of my army papers.

We had been scheduled in such a fashion as to arrive at Seattle airport, via military bus from FT. Lewis, Washington in the early morning hours while the airport traffic was almost void of civilians. The travelers primarily made up of soldiers returning from Vietnam and, you guessed it, new meat for the war offering, FNG's (Fucking New Guy). The Army has an acronym for just about everything as you are beginning to understand. As I'm sure that most reading this know, or possibly remembers the Government's plan to have soldiers avoid civilians whenever possible, was well thought out during the later years of the war. I never passed through an airport during my tenure with the Army that I didn't witness at least one incident started by a civilian to ridicule or embarrass a soldier with the usual slur of "baby killer", or "how many people did you kill? Usually a single soldier in uniform, not a group of two or more! I witnessed a single serviceman easily handle several civilians on one occasion with fellow servicemen rallying to fend off other troublemakers interested in joining the fray. We were told to refrain and remember who we were because we were in uniform.

At this point, there was absolutely nothing to gain, however when going, one might consider a chance to defer his torment by a short time while being raked over the coals by superiors that would yell and threaten worse, but still send you expediently on your way as you ask "What are you going to do, send me to Vietnam?".

After I checked in and bought my ticket, I walked over to the nearest bar and took a seat to have a beer and cheeseburger (the most dreamed about food while in country). Mine and June's all time favorite treat and the food I really dreamed of, was a Gino's Giant, fries and mocha shake. Anyway, at a small table nearby, I overheard a sergeant pumping three new kids full of his war stories and trying to scare the shit out of them (at 24, I felt like a sage Grandpa, a feeling that followed me even until I actually was one). Having either finished his drink or pleased that he had terrified three young soldiers, the sergeant left the table. I could hear most of the concerned conversation of the remaining three and turned toward them asking them to join me at the bar.

They looked at each other and then the most worried of the three came over and asked me, how bad is it? I bought them a beer and asked them to calm down, confirming that I had overheard the whole thing and that for whatever reason, felt he was just trying to scare them. Remember, I had just gotten paid in cash, so I could act like the big spender and hopefully the big brother, because I had already paid cash for my ticket.

It was a routine that a lot of seasoned soldiers did to new people in country, until they accepted that the guys were getting it, or until the next new guy came, whichever occurred first. Others tried their best to separate themselves from the new people for various reasons. Maybe they had lost friends recently or worse, often, and they just didn't want to keep doing it over and over, it being much easier to just not make new friends. The logic was that FNG's were most likely to be the next casualty, because chances increased as they had the least ability to react and perform when the stimulus required and obviously knew the least about everything facing them.

And finally, they were once FNG's and probably treated the same way, so it was basically payback or a personal method of training the individual to get his shit together quickly or go home in a body bag. Getting your shit together referred to having loose shit, a double meaning that the FNG didn't have his wits and skill set together yet, or the fact that the required daily malaria pills, caused loose bowels, especially when Cherry, and beginning the dosage, flaky shit, or condensed start to finish, loose shit = blown up (scattered) shit, FNG = body bag. I personally did not like that type of treatment, did not disparage a new guy, and tried to stop it when I could, but these young men at the airport bar were getting this bullshit before they even left the states, and I was offended and disturbed by that.

I told them that I would let them know what it was like, as things were slowing down and troops were withdrawing and that the other sergeant and I were examples of that, in having received early outs. I gave them a brief rundown of the action now being primarily in the Northern I Corp, and told them they would most likely go to the 101st as that was the predominate division still operating in the hot areas, knowing they were infantry. I told them that it can be as bad as you make it yourself, so go into it with as positive an attitude as you can muster.

Finally, I told them what I was told by my uncle, a full colonel, before I left. Keep your head down, listen to what the senior guys tell you, don't do anything stupid, remember your training and don't volunteer for anything, especially LRRP's (Long Range Reconnaissance Patrol). We talked a little longer before my flight and I believe I eased their minds at least a little and I'm sure a few more drinks aided the cause. Nothing or no one could make them unafraid! I remember it being the most empty, lonesome and fearful feeling in the world the previous year, and still do, it paling only to when I lost my lover, June.

The next time I had someone ask me that question, believe it or not, was three years later, when my Mom and my grandmother asked me if I had killed anyone while there. I will explain that confrontation as I evolve the story, as I was lucky enough to have two 18-22 year olds ask me during the last fifteen years, both doing research for college courses on the Vietnam era. I spent several hours on the phone and in person with both, a young daughter of a co-worker friend, and a young male friend of one of my grandsons, respectively.

I was somewhat nervous at the beginning of the first discussion, mostly done via email, but knowing the young lady very well, eased through the discussions. I hadn't discussed it much in the earlier years, but I am always thinking both consciously and subconsciously about that part of my life, as I continue to add information obtained from reading and conversations with other vets. As I began responding to the questions, mostly of social content, I was able to flow right through and it reflected for me, both older feelings I held and revised feelings as represented by newer opinions in my life as well as newer reflections as discerned from my readings and media.

The later example was with the young man that was the approximate age as I had been at deployment. It was easy to sit with and look at him to relate how I felt with a new wife, him being a single young man in college, me being drafted into war and him having the choice, as his brother had recently enlisted in the Army. Coincidentally, we were able to watch one of the newer episodes of a new Vietnam war documentary by Ken Burns.

I could and did use that episode as talking points while answering his questions which were all across the spectrum compared to the earlier session with the young woman. Both experiences were wonderful for me. I had more questions asked by these two young people who could have been my grandchildren, than I have ever had from anyone, including my family and friends. Of course it was uplifting and a good release for me and I have always hoped that I was able to help them achieve a good grade from their assignments because it had given me some relief to express myself without any worry or compulsions.

Many of us kept the majority of our experiences to ourselves while deployed in most cases, but especially after returning home, at least in the initial stages of our return and for much longer time frames in other cases. Theoretically, using common sense, the longer a person holds things inside, the worse things will be when forced to deal with them or conceivably may erupt negatively if not dealt with. It was a new era for combatants, as every new war is, not knowing what might develop in your body and mind as you try to reclaim your life which has been put on hold.

Following my return from Ft. Lewis in my first Boeing 747 flight, which was as spectacular as I thought it might be, partially because the seven of us vets in first class were living high on the hog. We were there all alone with two stewardesses (not flight attendants at that time) enjoying drinks and first class appetizers and dishes we had never heard of before, but enjoyed immensely, except for the pigs feet. We were treated wonderfully and thanked for our service by the crew and absolutely nil questions were asked. We had our own bathrooms up there and the curtains were drawn, so we never commingled with the civilians as described earlier. The captain and crew came back and spoke with us as we disembarked and entered the terminal through a gateway first in line ahead of those in coach.

Of course I was only looking for June, who I had left at the terminal gate in Hawaii just two months earlier, but saw my brother first, then Mom, my sister-in-law and a good friend. They all hugged and greeted me and I asked where June was, and my Mom said that her boss would not let her leave work and come pick me up.

I was totally deflated at the fact that she couldn't take part of a day off and greet me, realizing that it was probably related to disdain for the war effort, but we hurriedly headed off from the terminal to the car. My Dad was on a trip, as their crews traveled with each charter group, usually one to two weeks on the road and three to six days at home, depending on the trips he was bidding. There were some war protests at the airport as they usually were, but I imagine because I was surrounded by my family and friends I was not taunted at all. I didn't have any luggage because I threw away everything I wore to Ft. Lewis and carried from Vietnam, rather than have any questionable contraband, a large deterrent threat to hold you for investigation if found, as we processed out. Better off taking nothing, rather than have a chance of being retained.

After we had loaded into the car and began driving, Lee driving, Mom in the front passenger seat, looked back and asked me to explain my ribbons, which took a quick thirty seconds. Not one person asked a question about my explanations, and no other question was asked of me other than the traditional how are you, how was the flight, how long did it take, etc. I asked some of those questions back to them and we exchanged other information about family and friends when Lee announced that they were having a welcome home party for me that night at his house since it was the weekend.

When we got to my parents' house I went up to my bedroom and changed and took a long shower, and flushed the toilet just for the fun of it, found some summer clothes and went downstairs to talk to Mom and wait for June. A few hours later, June walked in and we greeted each other and sat and talked for a while until we went up and got ready for the party. Remember, we were in Mom's home.

She didn't have any hard questions for me either, and come to think of it, didn't while we were in Hawaii on R & R. I didn't really expect too much of that from her though, because I wrote her so often and tried to keep her up on everything, as instructed by the wise E-8 when first arriving in Vietnam, I had not told her anything that would cause her concern. My Uncle, however had told both of my parents to give me room and not to ask many hard questions and advised them that it would be very unusual for me to tell them very much at all, and knowing my personality, probably nothing. His final warning, that they would probably never know what I went through while there, and not to press me.

I always wondered if he had contacted any higher up friends of his, about me while I was in country, because I knew he was following my progress in Ft. Benning, because I got word from a drill sergeant that my uncle was going to attend our final PT (Physical Training) the next day. He followed Lee's and my football and wrestling career closely, as he played college ball as his two sons did as well, his oldest behind Lee and I at U of D. I was a nervous wreck that I wouldn't perform to his satisfaction and embarrass him and myself and my Mom's sister, but luckily for me, he didn't show. Whew!! All of that concern and I passed easily, scoring high on everything but the mile run, my albatross.

I will mention will a little pride, and shift of gears, that during my NCO training we ran everywhere we went, sometimes miles between classes and weapons ranges, and our training company CO (Commanding Officer), joined us in the base PT group Run For Life, which resulted in five mile plus runs after evening mess, reportedly running more than 500 miles, during my NCO training. Of course it was mandatory and by the end of that training cycle I had been able to achieve what runners call, their "second wind", after feeling exhausted and continuing the run to feel refreshed with new vigor. After the first night of capturing that high, I cruised through the runs, until I started running again years later as my son was pulling into his athletic prowess and I didn't want to be left too very far behind. I never achieved the high again, ever, and I did slip far, far behind my sons capabilities.

A few weeks after my welcome home party, we were in our first apartment as husband and wife, working and moving on. June continued with her career at the hospital and I began my continuation courses at the university and working second shift in the local Chrysler auto assembly plant, converted to Plymouth and Dodges after being originally built in the 1940's as an army tank plant.

I moved into a management training position training hard core employees (welfare recipients, exprisoners, and veterans unable to find work), roughly one year later. The "hard core" trainees were entering a career in the large factory, from the service, prison or welfare roll and unemployment. We taught them how to maintain bank accounts and personal finances while learning how to budget a solid income, coming from a minor fixed income, physically adjusting to the rigor of working on the line and learning how to communicate and care for their families while in that environment. The graduates of the program showed a significantly better performance average over off the street hires. The job was funded by the federal government and was a prototype operation in several of Chrysler's plants, attempting to show the correlation of improved performance with proper indoctrination education, which increased production.

I had spent a little over a year working in the trim department on various jobs, but primarily on the instrument panel line for Plymouth and Dodge and was very grateful for the opportunity and pay increase, all a result of my performance and conduct, per my foreman.

I thoroughly enjoyed my job, had a great boss and three other individuals that I worked with, who took me under their wing and brought me up to speed quickly. I started mostly with clerical work as I was an excellent typist, had good attitude and was eager to learn, assisting in their training and teaching routines in a few weeks.

After a month or so, I started making some minor corrections in my bosses reporting while typing and a few months later he asked me if I wanted to try and pull his monthly recap report together to send to corporate. I jumped at the chance and after a few corrections over a couple months, he told me that I could continue on my own with his final review, which afforded him enough time to spend a few hours of the day with his son at a local retail shop he owned.

A few months after starting in the new job, June became pregnant with our first child and Shannon was born that August, 20, 1973, a strong healthy beautiful little girl. June and I were on cloud nine and continued moving right along in our jobs as her Mom helped her through the six week leave from work and stayed on for a few months as we developed our routines.

A year later or so later during the summer, the first national fuel shortage hit the economy hard and most car plants shut down for changeover as they did each summer and carried all assembly workers on temporary layoff for several months afterward. We worked through the layoff, but because of the additional shutdown and primarily the fuel shortage, the government also shut down the training program permanently as hiring was curtailed.

That meant I would have to return to the factory at an elevated status, but they had no foreman jobs open because things were slower, so I returned to the line. I moved around a bit as they adjusted crews and gained a lot of experience working on the seat line, body shop welding, and final line at the seat installation station.

After the transition, I began having what I thought to be sinus problems. I had been working to improve our new yard quite a bit as it was seeded and lightly landscaped as new lots are. I worked night shift then, so made a doctor appointment with my long time physician and neighbor. He couldn't find anything wrong as mentioned previously, but because of my symptoms which included headaches, malaise, night sweats and aches in my back, he had me tested because he thought I might have carried malaria back with me or had a relapse of a mild case. The results of the test were negative and I was feeling a lot worse, so he checked with Chrysler and ran some allergy tests because it was somewhat common to have allergies in the cushion plant as well as the welding plant because of the materials required in the assembly process.

Again, the tests were negative, so he sent me to an ENT specialist where he took one look up my nose, and noticing the Afrin in my shirt pocket asked me if I had one by the bed, in the car and at work? I smiled and said yes, and he pronounced me "hooked on Afrin" and said the only way off was cold turkey and I had to buck up and throw them all away.

June and I tossed every bottle that night and I hoped I would get better, but other than my nasal passage opening up as the days passed, I became more tired and depressed about, who knows what, I just didn't feel right and June and I started arguing and not getting along all the time. After a short time, they shut down again because things were continuing to slow because of the gasoline situation and they began announcing layoffs, but I was ok for now, having built up over two years seniority. At least I was finally free of the Afrin fixation and was breathing lot easier. I knew I had at least the next several months or so off until they started the line again and was being paid 90% of my normal pay between unemployment pay and union subsidy pay, so the money was ok, but I was in a bad state of mind.

My favorite grandmother was up from South Carolina visiting my Mom, so I decided to go over there one day and talk to my own personal shrink. Mom and she knew the situation I was in and had talked to her sister, the colonels wife to ask her about my uncle's experience with his Vietnam troops and their returns. PTSD was a long way from being discussed at that time, but of course we now know I had the symptoms.

We began a normal family discussion and it quickly morphed into a bad scene. Mom and her mom were both very religious and started asking me to go see the preacher and ask for help and started asking me what was wrong with me, raising their voices and asked me if I had killed anyone. I flew off the handle at them and told them it was none of their business what I did and asked what right did they have to ask me personal things like that and that I couldn't talk about it at all.

Nothing I could offer would help them understand where my head was. They asked me again about religion and if I prayed over there and did I still pray. I flipped out again and told them that I went to Sunday services in the beginning when I could, but stopped because the Chaplain was always talking about how god was going to be helping us over the "gooks", because we were Christians, and they were heathens who did not believe in the true god. Many of the viet cong were Catholic and there were Catholic orphanages all over the place, but to him they were all "gooks" and heathens.

I sat through a few of those sermons and thought how nonsensical all that sounded to me, as I was sure those guys were praying to keep from getting killed and wounded as well. What made the god we prayed to, any more likely than theirs to answer their prayers as opposed to ours? I thought back to all the football, baseball, wrestling matches, when I had prayed to be able to do well while playing, and had always felt a little guilty. But I kept asking to get a hit, a TD, a pin, etc., not wanting to fail or disappoint myself or others.

The three of us continued for a while longer, but I was so upset during the ordeal that I don't remember all of the details, only that I was extremely distraught, angry and worried about how I was acting toward them and talking to them.

My grandmother told me she loved me and I just looked at her. My mother did the same thing and tried to hug me and I just froze. My lifelong favorite person in the world, my grandmother, asked me if I loved she and Mom again. I snarled at them that I would explain how I felt about them very clearly, and proceeded to tell them, "Yes I love you both, but you could both die tomorrow and I would be sorry and upset, but be over it the day after."

They started crying and hugging each other and my grandmother said "Bub, (my family name Bub or Bubba because my brother called me Bubba as he couldn't say brother when I was born) you don't mean that son!", always son when she was serious with me. I told them "Yes I do, it's the way I feel right now."

They left me alone for about a half hour and came back saying they wanted to help and asked if I could continue to talk about any of it. I had calmed down a bit and tried to explain that it had been difficult and lonely losing friends over there, and it ate you up for too long under the circumstances, because you had to have your wits about you to keep going.

You were always scared of everything, lonely, afraid to be wounded or killed and the only thing we continued doing was throwing up shields to prevent getting close to others. To my knowledge, most of us did it. It didn't work, but you learned very fast to not get emotional, at least not show it in the open, but at night , alone, it took its toll. You were always told to shut up and suck it up if you did talk about it. There were several universal phrases generated and passed through the GI's throughout the country, that somewhat sums things up. "Don't mean nothin'", whenever a complaining statement was made or a negative event happened, also a song by Nancy Sinatra, "Ain't no big thing", self explanatory, "I heard that", any negative or good information, "What are they gonna do, send us to Vietnam?", when threatened with discipline, and "Sheeeit!", a statement in itself.

I had never consciously even thought about those feelings since being home, truly. The more I thought, the more I saw what was helping cause problems between June and I. That realization of course, was not immediate, but began to materialize as time and problems progressed over the years.

I feel that I had shown her very little personal emotion since I came home. Not on purpose, and I didn't even see myself doing it. I apologized for the words to my mom and grandmom, but I didn't retract them, and told them I was trying to describe how I felt, that it was my problem to solve and I could only do that by myself.

I was not the only young man who lost their religion while in Vietnam, as I knew quite a few who admitted to me similar feelings, as well as determined from the books I've read, documentaries I've watched and people I've talked with. Others had the opposite reaction, and felt that they found their religion while there, the no atheists in a foxhole types. When a young man was dying in that war, he more often than not, called for his mother or his wife or girl, not his god and most often a chaplain was no where near, but a friend or medic was. I believe that has probably always been the case because of the youth of the combatants, like me, almost forced to go to church as a young person, not by choice and rewarded if I behaved during the sermons.

I do remember slightly revolting at my parents when I started working and they required me to tithe 10% of my meager earnings and began asking them if they tithed 10% and got their reasons why it wasn't quite that much, and asking
myself questions about my real feelings on religion. I realized I had been slowly withdrawing from it, most likely because I wasn't playing sports any more and felt guilty asking for good things for myself, while I was beginning to realize the fact there were many others in real need and later in life, my best friend always telling me that no matter how bad you think you have it, just look around and you will find someone worse off, there always was as far as I have been able to see, even now.

I fear that many people primarily or only believe they must believe, in order to have a chance for a life after death, if there is any such thing and/or maybe because they are afraid to die, afraid of the unknown, that many appear to believe they know. I talked often to my Mom about that from the time I came home until she died. I told her that I couldn't understand her being so afraid of leaving this world if she had such a better place ahead and she could be with all of her family, and that I would be there soon enough, or before her. I said that I understood why she had her beliefs, as I do with everyone, and am happy that they take comfort in their beliefs, but I don't happen to share them, and never had any comfort in that philosophy. If they need them to feel complacent in life, then so be it.

I've been disappointed too many times in my life to believe that these things were preordained and happened for a reason to be known later. I'm a see it to believe it person, but I do believe in some spiritual things I have experienced alone and with others and openly and fondly speak of them. I'm for everyone having the right to believe in anything they need in order to get through this life with as much peace and love in their heart and mind that is possible. To me, that is what it's all about, handle it any way you need to in order to be complacent.

I have often wondered he often feel that life itself might even be the Hell, so dreaded after death, and maybe death is true peace, the end. To me, all that matters, is that no one should be judged or persecuted for whatever they believe. If there are people that don't want to associate with me because of what I believe, that is fine with me, but I will never, stop my association with anyone strictly because of their beliefs on this nor any matter, as everyone has the right to be their own individual person, and should be in charge of their beliefs.

I went home to June and we briefly discussed what had gone on at Mom's house that afternoon. After dinner and putting Shannon to bed, we went to bed and continued the discussion. I told her exactly what I had told them verbatim and she started asking me similar questions and criticizing me for hurting their feelings. She asked me if I felt the same about she and Shannon, and I said no, that it was different with them, but she surely sensed that it wasn't too different.

I guess I was somewhat distant to everyone that I was naturally close to, but did not realize it. This is about three years after my return and we had never talked about anything other than stories and people I had written about in my self censored letters. I started crying and apologized for not showing her the type of feelings and emotion she deserved, and told her I would try and change that back to the way it used to be, but was skeptical.

She kept probing and I began explaining one operation I was on early in my tour and got to some very gory parts when she stopped me, and asked "why is that still bothering you now, that was years ago and it shouldn't still bother you?" I had no real answer and just stared at her shaking my head as we both fell to sleep, me crying, never finishing the story and in the morning she went right on to work as usual.

That night when she came home, things were pretty much the same as they had been. I loved her just as much as I always did, more than anyone ever, but I couldn't say it and express it the way I used to, which she needed and didn't know why or what was the matter with me. I know these things now, but had no realization of them at that time.

Time moved a little forward and we both tried to improve the situation but made very little headway. I believe now, that I had caused her to regress toward my position by treating her the way I did, but I was not aware of that at the time either.

We started thinking I should leave Chrysler because things didn't look or sound good because of my health, the economy and I wanted to try to find a position I could grow in, as that seemed to be gone at Chrysler. I began applying for a lot of local jobs without success and finally answered an ad in the newspaper for a manufacturing consultant to travel Monday through Friday. June and I talked and off I went in a few days to Philadelphia and my interview. In had the qualifications and got along well with my interviewer, a partner in the international company based in Chicago.

I was soon hired, and within a few weeks scheduled to leave on a Sunday to begin my traveling, consulting career with great hopes and anticipation, but dreading that I had to leave June and Shannon for a week at a time. I had no idea how that was going to work out, nor did June. We discussed it for those few weeks and thought that we could make the most of it because we loved each other and Shannon and had to make it work, regardless of the problems it presented, so we tried.

The effects of war on everyone, especially participants and families are lifelong. They don't just disappear or stop when you come home. Just as we always remember our first kiss, our first true love, our first death, our first fight, our children's' births, our true hardships along the way, the effects of war cycles through our lives again and again. That is one reason I think and write in this style, where subjects change, but life continues because familiar feelings appear suddenly and often bring change.

The declarations of war and the effect on the citizens of warring nations is always extreme. It is my contention that every war before yours was more difficult than yours. I'm not speaking for those combatants that had horrific injuries, because no matter what war or other tragedy you might suffer, one can be as devastating as the other without regard to when it happened.

To the WIA's (Wounded In Action), whether your leg is blown off by a booby trap, a cannon ball, hacked off with a sword, sawed off by a field doctor after a gruesome wound or other cause, I would imagine they suffered much the same at the time of the injury. The big differences come immediately after the injury and how quickly they were attended to, on average.

Obviously you can't cherry pick all of the conditions and parameters of the incident, because you could make no true comparison. You have to look at the operational procedures, job skills of the team and individual, average or similar weather, and other indices in order to determine how one faired immediately, short term and long term. As far as those that are KIA (Killed In Action), I think the only difference is that the further you go back in time, many more died from what we would consider non life threatening wounds, because they received little or no help on the battlefield and succumbed for various reasons as simple as exposure, loss of blood, shock, or never made it to an aide station, if they even existed.

Considering these circumstances and walking backwards from one generational war to the next, many things have changed for the positive, which produce an improvement in treatment and care. I will not try to describe incidents for specific injuries from current battle grounds or those throughout history, but just utilize common sense to illustrate my beliefs.

Common sense has been the defining tool for me since I knew of it and discovered I had an ability to utilize it while making conscious decisions for my own good and that of others. I talk about it often and have used it throughout my life, in all facets of my life and placed a very high value on it and those able to manifest it in order to traverse through life. In my final three jobs, thirty-one years total, I hired scores of employees and looked for common sense indicators above education, in many cases. It rarely failed me and I have always tried to teach employers and employees of its value and feeling of accomplishment in using it.

I believe that it is the basis of the conscience and will delve into that further on in this writing. I also gave great consideration to all minorities in the workplace including women, veterans, and athletes, because of their focus, dedication and teamwork, in an effort to integrate the immediate workforce. I always ranked employees by job and performance in my mind, which I learned as a great management tool during my consulting career, and worked toward helping the best of them, work toward taking my job or other lead jobs, for my good as well as my company.

Obviously, technology is the largest of the improvements. Just looking at the medical knowledge, techniques, blood clotting agents, battlefield equipment and medicines continuing to improve significantly as we move forward. Diagnostic equipment, deployment of specialists, procedures for traumatic injuries, head and brain injuries, and medical histories of treatments continued to improve and I assume always will.

Transportation technology for evacuating wounded combatants jumped exponentially with the advent of the helicopter in Korea and continues to improve with the changing technology. Will the WIA be beamed to an aide station somewhere in the future, or will we be civil and smart enough to use our common sense and not kill each other as needlessly by then.

After technology, I would say that operational tactics follow closely behind, however it is hard to isolate that without technology improvements and which came first, the chicken or the egg? We have certainly improved our chances of lowering casualties by not wearing red coats and lining up five deep, which seemingly allows any somewhat aimed shot, friendly shot, even single load, to hit a victim, or a cannon ball bouncing through the ranks taking out multiple aggressors, like a bowling ball barreling through pins. It is quite easy to see how the technological improvement in equipment and weapons drives a change in tactics like taking cover in trenches and dispersing into fortified bunkers when machine guns came into use.

Assaulting thousands of young men up cliffs with modern weapons and fortifications in front, above and below them, while their back is to the sea, is a conundrum I haven't been able to fit into the time frame, but certainly didn't encompass much common sense, but maybe desperation or worse, fatalism. After reading about those invasions in history, I hoped that nothing like those battles would ever happen again. To my chagrin, they did happen, but luckily on a smaller scale and are hopefully in a diminishing trend.

Overhead cover, fox holes, steel helmets and flak vests certainly saved a lot of lives when lobbing weapons such as hand grenades and mortars became common on the battlefield. Artillery begat artillery duals in addition to dropping rounds on infantry, cavalry or stationary targets, and so on. It seems that as weapons continue to evolve and are more powerful and have greater range, the tactical changes turn to mostly developing defensive weapons. Heavy caliber machine guns and RPG's (Rocket Propelled Grenades), in addition to rifles became a deadly weapon against helicopters in the beginning, adding booby traps and ambushes on LZ's added new techniques.

Later and in mountainous areas where concealment was amplified, anti aircraft weapons were used for low flying fighters and bombers and pressed into service as viable additional weaponry for helicopters. Newer rocket technology evolved into shoulder fired missiles, and heat sensing missiles for high flying bombers. Surface to air, air to surface, air to air missiles all evolving as the improvement of flight and rocket technology improved.

It seems that in the earlier conflicts technology pushed tactics and as time marched on it becomes muddied, which pushes which. Is there any battlefield tactic now that can withstand, let alone defeat the newest technologies such as remote control drones and other newer equipment , or will it come down to who initiates the first or the largest nuclear attack.

There are many defensive weapons manufactured and sold to many countries, touted as sufficiently capable to counter ballistic missiles, but they have not been proven effective to any sufficient degree on live targets. The initial successes in the early 1990's were greatly exaggerated and even erroneous from what I remember reading and using my first hand experience in war reporting, to the extent of false claims of knock downs to likely shooting down allied aircraft. Let alone, the natural law of whatever goes up must come down, somewhere! Current adversaries claim to have the perfect system, but again, not sufficiently proven. Easy to taut perfection testing on your own weapons, much harder to ever prove until it may be too late as we have seen with our own tests, with questionable positive results, yet countries scramble to purchase.

Will wars end because of a standoff between nations racing to achieve the best technology to be first and the deterrent, or will vast populations be destroyed as the result? Could there possibly ever be enough defensive systems available, with their inadequacies of countering speed, accuracy, destructive force, and quantity, to protect any and all positions? I don't see that possibility happening as I can only assume the expense of those defensive systems less important to the more powerful nations than the productions of the offensive weapons. Much easier to hit a fixed target. The race is on for how many totally destructive weapons, not defense.

On that note maybe we should explore the accuracy of valid wartime statistics and information. This is one area that I believe we might be headed in a reverse direction as to credibility very quickly and not just as it occurs in wars.

As war continues to produce decreasing numbers of lives lost by warriors over fixed time spans, it appears the cost in national treasures could be increasing in possibly exponential amounts. The cost of these new technologies is extravagantly large and those expenses can convert to and become a monstrous source of income in trade with less industrial and capable nations, producing gigantic profits for the manufacturing countries. The manufacturers increase prices because the government will push that additional cost off to the international buyers with bigger profits.

There will be less worry about government costs as that is born by taxpayers. The increased government profits will be squandered by individual owners and stockholders for who knows what end game, as history shows and will not be passed on to the lower layers of taxpayers or workers. The countries capable of the technology and manufacturing will soon become saturated in inventory for national requirements and will seek to sell them to those other less fortunate countries seeking protection from more capable enemies, via fear mongering, saber rattling and desire of increasing defense capabilities, allowing more and more dangerous weapons across the world creating a cascading effect.

Slowing down the wealth growth, let alone ending it will not be deemed acceptable by manufacturers and owners, nor the governments of the countries. More wars will begin or be prolonged in order to keep the profits flowing. As more countries stockpile the more impressive and expensive weapons, the threat to loss of human life grows dramatically, if not by combatants, but by collateral damage victims as a simple compounded result of more weapons in the hands of unqualified and uncaring warriors, especially hostile regimes.

As long as the powers to be can maintain the coolness of control, wisdom and restraint of pushing the nuclear buttons, less soldiers will die and the money will grow. Without wars continuing or beginning somewhere on earth, those requirements will end. My guess is that we will continue to see growth of those who choose to be hawkish or as I like to call them war mongers.

It is much more harsh but more direct and realistic of what history always produces. There never seems to be a loss of potential threats to make that generation of officials in every part of the world see the possible need for war, thereby commanding the need to continue the weapon stockpiles and development.

Better than energy to drive wealth, as energy is used by all and most contribute to its development or at least have the potential, thereby holding prices more steady, because the whole world needs it. Whoever builds and sells the top weapons, which they won't let other countries participate in, will always be the wealthiest, and more importantly, those in control of who dictates conflict and controls the resulting monetary rewards.

Will technology create stalemates where even weapons in outer space may be neutralized or matched, to no advantage? Does weapon technology then shift toward weapons to defend against or even attack the unknown, but perceived possibility of armies of aliens from space, just to keep the technology and money flowing? I guess that we can always create unseen enemies. What is certain, is that that source of national wealth cannot and will not just disappear, nor will these mighty weapons

The rich will get richer as history confirms, but how rich does one nation, one group of people, or one person need to be? Humans have been battling humans since the beginning, with no complete stoppage and none foreseen, while weapons stockpiles continue to grow in order to grow the wealth of the defense companies and countries.

Yes, we claim victories and treaties, but continue to push others to the brink of war by whatever reason we can convince our countrymen. Every nation is involved to a lesser or greater degree, based on those original reasons and causes for war.

In these somewhat harsh and certainly dire projections I am forecasting as a possibility, armed combatant casualties would decrease, which might somewhat stabilize the recruitment of armies, but collateral deaths and damage is most likely to increase proportionately with the power and quantity of the weapons. These factors are increased again exponentially, with the use of nuclear weapons.

What do we do to avoid these results if these situations are realized, or do we at some point find another way to work as one people and save the world and human race? Why not stop the weapons unilaterally and increase the technology with peaceful aspirations and the belief that the world can work together in order to make more equality to all levels of modern society, share the wealth and even things out for everyone. I told you I was optimistic. We had made progress, now we slide backwards.

I begin with these statements and questions to explore some of the braggadocio achievement hypotheses, to look at the reasons wars might originate. Wars traditionally began over lust for power and control, followed by greed for territory, values and treasures or nationalistic goals, claims of perfect races and destruction of others.

Throw in some religious persecution, human rights, pure hate, and even the occasional woman, and you create the tender for a possible world sized forest fire. How did we arrive at this point in such a short period of time in this human civilized society, compared to the timeframe of man, a nano second as related to geological time?

I'm not sure where it might have begun, but I can use common sense and self experiences, to conjure up some possible reasons. Whatever those reasons above, either all or in part, that greed and desire became an absolute must for each side. In modern historical examples, sometimes devious confrontations were involved in the decision to go to war, over portrayed and some of which were possibly known about before hand, coordinated, inflated, conflated and even possibly created for the desired effect. Without listing specific facts to cast blame, I will list some examples, realizing that I am stating them not as fact, but contributing actions for cause, in no particular order. Assassination of country head, manipulation of proof of weapons of mass destruction, previous knowledge of sneak attacks, false reports of sinking of ships and false attacks, conceived threats of communist incursions, incursions over sovereign borders, ignoring and/or downplaying active intelligence, fear mongering to exacerbate fear into assertive action, etc.

A beginning like that can only grow into other exaggerations, massaging and outright fabrication. The desire of those in charge, on all sides, is to win in a non-challengeable way. To do that, positive results must be achieved and more importantly, reported to the constituents of the warring sides to uphold support and continue support for, and approval of war funds.

If things really are going well, factual information can be reported, but better news, especially early in the campaign, could enhance the support in many ways.

If things appear to be slipping the wrong way, information might be massaged so as not to loose the interest and support of the people , thus the treasures. A very hard uphill road may lie ahead when a slow or encumbered beginning is conceived and then conveyed. Not a good way to start a war, therefore both sides claim to be on a winning path in the initial stages, or nothing definitive is reported at all.

What continues as the war continues, reminds me of the old parable my grandmother used to tell my brother and I while growing up. "Oh what a tangled web we weave, when first we practice to deceive." Most of us have started down that road a time or two, but hopefully found out that the further you continued, the more tenuous it became, so hopefully, you righted the ship and felt a sigh of relief.

Some of us most likely continued down the proverbial road a time or two and suffered some harsh results or worse. Those who have travelled that road to fruition, probably still have bad dreams of them or at least bad thoughts nagging at their conscience, and problems remembering everything as told to be able to continue the spin, therefore the longevity of life of the web.

The problem is that the beginning starts the benchmarks for the remainder, which begin at the end of the previous war, if you won. If you lost, you might be tempted to start with higher bench marks and set more rewarding goals, create new indicators, or choose other choices of resolve instead of war.

The length of the war probably helps determine the rapidity of achieving these goals. As wars progress, we have historically found increasing methods of disbursing the good news and likely the downplay of not so good news. This information is controlled to a large extent, as are the operational techniques of the war, by technology.

Just look how technology changed from the Civil War to the first Gulf War. Official army reporting via pencil and paper, sometimes telegraph, word of mouth and news print, even occasional photographs, to full modern media blitzes with imbedded reporters in many units sometime reporting live, which possibly presented slight security problems. The lesson there, censorship and delayed reports, not by the media, but the authorities. The media needs to report the truth always, but there do arise occasions that it should be delayed so as not to disclose operational actions on an as occurring basis. Delayed, but not ignored or altered.

Radio and telephone use began in the early 1900's but were obviously crude and limited for reporting essential information from unit to unit and directing support function. As war technology increased, the communication capabilities did also, as did the available use to the ground units personnel. In the Vietnam war, field units fully equipped with radios available for each unit size down to squad and even fire team in some cases, and snipers, observation posts and listening posts had temporary custody of units while deployed.

The radio became the spear point for the on demand, as it occurred reporting of the new combat statistic gathering apparatus. While entire units could be employed in many AO's (Areas of Operation) at the same time, units from battalion and up had TOC's (Tactical Operation Center) on a fire base or base camp in the immediate vicinity which reported via landline and radio or teletype to upward units. The operating units communicated constantly up, down and across the organizational chart, but up and down continually, reporting location, direction of march and situation, and logistical hookups on an ongoing basis depending on unit procedures.

Cross organization commo was also used as needed for support functions such as artillery, medivac/dust-off and helicopter air support, and fixed wing air support and cover. NDP's (Night Defensive Positions) were called in every night after dark as units settled in for the night and posted and relayed to support units in order to coordinate H & I (Harassment & Interdiction) fires during the night for disruptive protection of locations pre marked and called in by each unit at strategic locations and times as well as illumination, as required.

Every unit commander down to platoon sergeant had an (RTO) Radio Telephone Operator carrying and maintaining a radio, extra batteries and long antenna weighing in excess of twenty pounds in addition to his normal combat load. Some enlisted squad leaders and recon squad leaders carried their own radios, again depending on unit operational procedures.

Communicating with loved ones at homes was limited to good old snail mail, however we only had to write FREE on the upper right corner of an envelope or any thing you could write on including a C ration box. We did also have a MARS (Military Auxiliary Radio System) stations set up in some communication rooms, whereby you could sign up and wait for an opportunity to "phone home" if an emergency or special circumstance, usually initiated by Red Cross, but not always.

MARS was a system of ham radio operators across the world that would attempt to relay and place a collect call to your loved one. Once registered you began your wait, which could be hours, and had to remember the 12 + hour time difference. If connected (about 50% chance), your loved one had to be instructed to say "over" every time they referred the call back to you and vice versa. I managed to get through two times, on weekends and middle of the night so my family would be awake during the day. By the time June or my Mom got through the first couple "overs", the allowed three minutes was over, but it was certainly was worth hearing their voices and probably much more rewarding for them.

One of my calls was made after I heard that an Airliner had crashed in Anchorage carrying troops to Vietnam. After further inquiry over radios, I discovered it was Capitol Airways, my Father's company, and I knew he was making as many trips over as possible to try and connect with me. Luckily for us it wasn't him, but terrible news for many families. They were certainly worth the wait of several hours and a half dozen failed attempts.

Talk about exponential advances, but nothing compared to the technology used now. I have mixed feelings about the newest technologies, whether it is good or bad to be able to stay in contact as closely as is available. I know it is better for peace of mind, but wonder about the mind of the service person during trying times. It is what it is, and time will tell.

As wars linger, so does the patience of the citizenry. Wars can certainly be too short, because the nations have to prepare for the deployment or battle for home turf, the manufacture or procurement of equipment, weapons, ammunition, and everything else in the constricting supply lines. All of that requires a war of some staying power and full treasure chests, as better profits must be produced over the costs of startup and depletion of treasures. Remember, the world revolves around the accumulation of money, in all forms. And of course the majority of those profits go to the upper echelon of that society, and conversely, most of the young men and women used to fight the war come from the lower echelons.

The decision makers help to control their own destiny in many cases, which has probably happened since the beginning of society and war. That doesn't mean that it should or shouldn't be that way, but that's a much larger undertaking than I'm prepared to further contemplate at this time. The right of the privileged goes all the way back to near the beginning per my common sense. Those with money, no matter what form, control the power to build the army, required or not and decide who is in the army.

You can begin to see the importance of good news reporting and statistics. Article One of our constitution provides for freedom of the press which allows more scrutiny in our reporting, especially compared to a dictatorship. However, the press, no matter how reputable and honest in any country, can not control the statistics nor guarantee they get a true look at all reports.

Going back to when most wars were gauged successful by the territory taken and held or lost, it was quite easy to ascertain where the lines of conflict areas began and ended and skirmish areas continued. Especially as technology grew and eyes were able be lifted by hot air, helium and finally flying aircraft and now, satellites.

Moving forward in history, the lines began to blur with the newer operational tactics and new available technical advances, combined with the battle terrain. These changes made the objective of taking territory a no starter, so they determined. However in Vietnam, that didn't prove to be correct when the NVA marched across the DMZ and through Cambodia and Laos, like Sherman's Civil War march through the South, after the US turned the war over to the RVN army, and congress cut off all support. What developed was a single Vietnam with no DMZ and new communist regime, very much different than results in Korea.

Small territorial areas of high ground and/or of strategic value to transportation infrastructure were prepared for construction and occupation. These areas were enclosed by perimeter defenses, developed for supporting facilities and troops, fortified and manned with support troops and equipment, as tactical units were dispersed to AO's to conduct search and destroy missions.

Ground/objectives were certainly taken during these operations, but usually not held for a long period of time before it was vacated, some immediately, others after fortifications were destroyed and thoroughly searched. Often these former objectives were obliterated by either artillery, air strikes, B52 arc-lights, and/or also seeded with solid pellets of CS gas (tear gas) on occasion. Very often, the enemy returned to their old hangouts and continued to pursue their enemy.

This was the beginning of a new progressional statistic reporting as related to success and failure. Many statistics were reported and compiled by the hour, day, week, month and year, by every fighting unit in the country. For the Army, squad to platoon, to company, to battalion, to brigade, to division, to corp, to army and finally combined with all of the other services and support units in country.

Of all of the statistics, the cherry on the top was the amount of US KIA vs Enemy KIA, US WIA and US MIA and Enemy prisoners, type, rank and injury. Obviously I am speaking about Vietnam directly now because this is where my primary interest and experience lies. It is noteworthy to mention also, that the authorities revised these methods as wars moved into the future due to considerable discrepancies, distaste of high numbers of casualties of friendly troops, and the developing ratios that became the measure of success or failure, later seen by the citizens as crass and less than acceptable.

Statistics of this nature are also very easy to generate as well as easy to compound errors in reporting. Everyone has probably played the parlor game of whispering a brief story from one person to the next completely around the room, I'm sure. We all know that the story is almost always unrecognizable when it gets to the end, often even changing the characters' names and gender. Consider how many steps these statistics pass to the final report. Look how errors may initiate and constrict or expand during just one line of communication.

Next, think about the confusion during and immediately after a fire fight or attack, and the horrific confusion, noise, screaming, distraction and mindset, let alone loss of and damage to the communication gear, and how all of that might relate to miscommunication of statistics, which is secondary to saving lives.

Now consider that each leader of each step is ultimately, at least partially, evaluated by his kill ratio. Then consider that there may be rewards such as cases of beer for specific numbers for the low end of the chain, to three day passes in country for mid levels of the reporting chain and so on. I will not extend it to the higher plateaus, but you certainly get the picture.

I'm not saying that this happened at every level, every time, but I am confident that it happened, not at every level from bottom to top every time, but sometimes at most of those levels and varying frequencies and often. Numbers hopefully, weren't grossly altered, but they were changed for a variety of reasons, as well as manipulated in many ways as well.

Obviously the US KIA and WIA internal numbers were accurate, as names, SSN's, types of wounds and type of contact were passed along the chain after location and medical requirements via secure methods, but the enemy numbers were, even at the lowest ranks, a prerogative, on occasion, and by the standards established requested or required to be a certain ratio, in order to be considered successful.

As a consultant, I would have used other ratios which used factual statistics within the friendly units. Statistics like friendlies killed, wounded, captured and missing against total munitions expended, meals issued, sorties flown, helicopters used and lost, and so on, in an effort to establish a reliable data base to compare against.

The growth of that data base would prove useful and could be worked against the actual goals being achieved or not and so on. The problem with those statistics is that you can not see how you are doing at the beginning of the war, but if they last as long as wars are now, what good information you would gather for future use.

And if the statistics were always used they could be adjusted in each war to the particulars of that war, therefore there would always be realistic data. A war needs instant assurance that it is working, but kill ratios certainly isn't it. Sure, you could count the enemy dead, blood trails, weapons, etc captured, but those are statistics in their own right and could be a comparison, but not a ratio as a goal because it is much to easy to manipulate, and as a thief that doesn't get caught, steals more until he does, so do the manipulators increase their success until found out and admonished, and not rewarded.

There were complaints of enemy KIA's too low, which drew orders to count body parts or each hand or foot as one body. There are reports of graves of enemy soldiers being dug up to count them as part of the total, creating a possibility that those enemy bodies had already been counted and left by US troops at the site, buried by their comrades and counted again.

If artillery, air strikes, helicopter gunship, or even navy battleship guns were used in an action, each of those units wanted credit for those kills. Determinations had to be made by type of wound and the source deduced by the men on the ground, flying overhead, or surmised by visible remains. Getting the picture? Sometimes math was used to divide the fatalities and give credit to each unit, sometimes more were added because the support unit had used "X" amount of munitions and thought it should have generated better results. There were a lot of errors in reporting but also a good bit of manipulation.

Possibly the same thing happened in reverse for the NVA, because the reports from their books seem to reverse those trends, but in quite different numbers, and then it begins a test of honor, and we can see that current history shows us how that works out in government. This is not an attempt to be critical but demonstrate the opportunities for the manipulation because of the desired results, a ratio of ours to theirs, as the final product is to demonstrate the characteristics of a successful war.

As the war continued and disharmony grew at home some decisions were made to limit artillery rounds during certain campaigns to "X" number per day per unit because most incoming munitions and supplies were beginning to shift to supply the South Vietnamese Army for the upcoming US drawdown, still years away from fruition. In addition to casualties there were many other statistics maintained on the same basis by support units. Helicopter sorties, airplane sorties, quantity of rounds of each type of artillery fired, navy guns fired, flame drops, agent orange barrels/sorties, helicopters retrieval's, medivac/dust-off extractions, types of helicopters and planes shot down, status of pilots, weapons, munitions, rice, intelligence, tunnels, bunkers captured or destroyed, and so on and so on.

Heavy combat casualties, and ordinance spent, artillery and aircraft, in one well known hill battle, flamed a directive from above to prevent heavy casualties from occurring during future contacts until the war was over. Even if it meant withdrawing, retreating, from battle earlier than necessary, again partially because of the Vietnamization of the war, material and action being passed from US to ARVN soldiers. The citizenry began to have enough of territorial gains that were immediately released back to the enemy after neutralized and fully decimated as well as too many friendly casualties and treasures lost.

I have read books recently published the past few years and even months, which continue to hold my attention and keep adding to my information bank. I can certainly relate to those books written about 1970-1971, in I Corp, by 101st unit members, both soldiers and pilots, as well as USAF pilots, both fighter and FACs (Forward Air Controller), and Marines from earlier tours because of working the same geographical locations where we relieved them. Those are the most interesting for me, however I like to follow the history of the war and the important engagements as well as certain units like the Big Red One, my uncle's division.

Most interesting to me because of the familiarity of the writing, but it is very interesting to understand the very different operating requirements and the vast changes in the terrain from the DMZ North to South and Coastal East to Laos and Mountains and Cambodia West and Delta South and East.

Battle gear varied from unit to unit such as required helmets and flak vests, to soft hats and no vests. Light web gear to full rucks with 40-70 pounds of various equipment depending on length of average stays in the field and logistics. Day treks from and to a fire base, to humping over a month before returning to a fire base or base camp and receiving periodic resupply by helicopter. Humps from fire bases to patrol the AO (Area of Operation), to helicopter combat assaults to LZ's (Landing Zones) hot or cold, prepped or not prepped.

Large unit Cavalry maneuvers with tanks and personnel carriers, while some rode and others walked, ever wary of the RPG's (Rocket Propelled Grenades) rocket trails.

Small recon squad clandestine rappelling insertions and sling extractions, from helicopter into and out of enemy territory including Cambodia, Laos, and the Demilitarized Zone and North with 4-10 per usual operation, lasting minutes to weeks or longer depending on contact with the enemy, some to never be seen or heard from again, some to be found killed and left in place.

Airmobile units varied in operations throughout the country largely dependent upon equipment and tactic variances, from Huey medivacs/dust-offs, troop carriers and gunships, to Cobra gunship red attack teams, Loach OH-1 observation and white attack teams, Loach and Cobra pink attack teams, Ranger courier and observation, Chinook CH-47 troop carriers, lift units, and flame drops, Sky Crane H-54 Target lift units and many more from other services.

Many unique combinations of helicopters and fixed wing aircraft incorporated unique procedures to produce fantastic results such as search lights, flare drops, infra red search and destroy teams and Agent Orange dusting flights. The famous AC-47 and AC-130's, Puff the Magic Dragon, and Spooky which provided close in ground support with flare drops, mini gun fire, automatic grenade fire, and cannon fire to often dominate and end many fire base attacks and separated ground unit attacks while providing many cavalry-like rescues of units in danger of being overrun.

Bomb damage assessments by ground units, helicopter solos or team searches, FAC and observation planes, Air Force, Navy and Marine fighter plane sorties, to determine effectiveness of arc-lights (bombing raids of the B52 Flights from Guam and Thailand), by counting dead and structural damage. Line units already in the field or inserted, often conducted air strike, naval bombardment and artillery damage assessments, primarily looking for bodies, body parts, wounded, equipment, intelligence data, caches and trails.

Personal preference of going without underwear and socks because you were out so long they began rotting off and to avoid jungle rot, to wearing underwear and changing socks frequently because of the water and mud and jungle rot. Monsoon season where you were wet continuously for days or weeks to the dry season with thick red dust that covered everything and left little red poofs of dust as you walked, and a day later might suck off a boot due to a heavy rain.

Being soaked with sweat constantly dripping from your helmet, hat, helmet or head with an GI OD (Government Issue Olive Drab) towel constantly around your neck to wipe you face, cover your head against mosquito attacks, cushion your shoulders from rucks and equipment, use as a pillow and serve as security blanket. Freezing at night during monsoons because you were never dry and a 30 degree drop in temperature, while still in the 60's, felt like winter.

Leaches stuck to your body and removed with lit cigarette or insect repellent, huge mosquitoes swarming, giant centipedes with poisonous bites, tarantulas, big black ants and smaller red fire ants. Small, two step pit vipers (two steps before you die), king cobras, pythons and everything in between. Monkeys and rock apes, giant lizards and elephants. Tigers and panthers sometimes visiting night ambush sites, mostly escaping, sometimes being blown to bits, sometimes taking a soldier and sometimes being killed by shock of the blast, soon to become a wound free, new rug for a unit commander.

But the rats, they were everywhere and some as big as house cats. I woke up one night with one on my chest and staring me red eye to brown. I was lucky enough to slap him away before he bit me, others weren't so lucky, while still others had contests to kill the most or in the most imaginative way. The most inventive method I saw, was the booby trapped ammo box, with tin of C ration peanut butter and blasting cap connected to a trip wire, one killed per trap, maybe a few more if lucky, with collateral damage.

The constant, sometimes daily, unpredictable attacks of incoming mortars, artillery, and rockets in the field to fire bases, to base camps and protected rear units were both frightful to debilitating for all, sometimes crippling or fatal for others. Bunkers were readily available but often not used because of being full of water, snakes, rats or as in my case the concept that it could hit the bunker as easily as where I presently sat, stood or resided. I remember diving into a bunker during my first rocket attack which was full of mud and water and never seeking another one, with the exception of a fighting bunker or sleeping bunker I was occupying at the time. There was always the fear of sapper infiltrations at night and full out assaults after incoming subsided.

Everyone took their turns on perimeter guard or resting/sleeping from the smallest ambush perimeter or listening post, fire base, base camp, to the largest and most secure rear area. Your first being a sleepless nerve frazzled night, thinking that you constantly see movement, swear you see a silhouette, keep checking your claymore clackers, wanting to ask for flares but afraid to be ridiculed, and waiting endlessly and sleepless for first light. The retaliating attack on a leader from a subordinate or subordinates for pushing too hard, making deadly errors or just unliked, usually accomplished with a grenade at night or while alone, even in a latrine, cruelly called a fragging, or mysteriously shot in the back during a firefight.

Tunnel systems that ran hundreds of yards stymied the imagination and enclosed caches of weapons, ammunition, rice, medical supplies, letters, communication equipment, generators, fans and sleeping quarters, with the occasional enemy soldier. Log and earth bunker complexes covering acres connected and protected by trenches, tunnels and spider holes (one man sniper pits with camouflaged mat covers) which you might not see until it was too late. Both types of fortifications could house multiple bed hospitals complete with running water and buried smoke stacks to conceal cooking fires. Snipers tied into trees with the utmost patience for the right shot with primary targets being officers, antenna identified radiomen, medics and point men. Some tunnels were found to be major complexes miles long and in some cases encroaching under friendly bases, found following the battle or war, and are now popular tourist sites.

There are even cases that some tunnels in conjunction with the Ho Chi Minh Trail network housed trucks and even elephants used in transporting material and hidden from air observers. Many of those trails and more inland trails were obscured from the air by patiently weaving overhead branches together when the natural canopy was not adequate to suffice.

The dreaded booby traps from simple toe poppers, punji pits, bouncing Betty, trip wire grenade/c ration can, devised to remove a foot or worse, impale an appendage or worse, bounce up waste high to explode and end your hopes of fatherhood or worse, and do bodily harm to anyone that trips the wire and his buddies within a few yards.

These and many others designed to maim or kill one or more servicemen, in order to feast on the soon to appear, target rich Huey dust-off helicopters, and gunships, or air cover. The inventive "mothers of all booby traps", the unexploded recovered ordinance such as mortar rounds, artillery shells, 250 to 500 pound bombs, and Claymore mines relieved from soldiers or captured and deployed against US troops, or chi-com claymores. These big boomers could destroy a whole fire team or squad, depending on how closely the soldiers were bunched, and could be trip wired or a command detonated ambush by an enemy soldier or soldiers near by.

These were the greatest fear of many servicemen, me included. I truly believed I would rather be dead than have to return home to my wife missing a foot, leg, both, or worse. There were often pacts made between foxhole buddies to ensure their friends received their wish, and were sometimes carried out as requested for selfish and unselfish reasons.

You have to remember that most of the grunts were 18 to 25, fresh out of high school or college, married or a special girl, usually athletic, proud and independent. I was scared shitless for lack of better words, the entire time I was in country that I might suffer such a fate, more than any other physical injury. I just could not bare the thought of going home to June minus anything, or go through the very harshly portrayed VA recuperative system.

The longer the war continued, the more stories in the news of these victims and their struggles in the VA hospitals back in the World. I can not hardly remember a day that did not contain multiple radio transmissions which were reporting one or more unit casualties from booby traps.

I personally had a friend from HS wounded severely by automatic weapon fire and returned to the World where he was treated long term and received his DD-214 and awarded disability status. He was diagnosed as never being able to gain total ability to walk, but luckily that changed as he continued to improve. He came to visit me at my parents' home after being discharged from the VA hospital, approximately one year before I was drafted. There weren't too many happy stories, but many horrible depictions of the sanitary conditions as well as the treatment.

"Born on the Fourth of July" is one movie that portrays an individual Marine from training to his being shot in the spine and paralyzed and follows him through the VA Hospital, back home, and traveling to Mexico and joining other wheel chair warriors in search of peace and camaraderie and finally demonstrating against the war. It is a heart wrenching story and there is a good amount of other documentation on the subject.

I personally stayed away from the VA medical facilities until I was diagnosed with Agent Orange related Multiple Myeloma and Chronic Kidney Disease 37 years later, with the exception of visiting my Father in Law in 1975 a few days before he died of an amputated toe related to diabetes. He was in a ward with about twenty other veterans and wasn't too happy about the care. That was the final time June and I saw him.

I was originally diagnosed with cancer in my home town civilian hospital and began immediately with my chemo treatments. I continued to work as much as possible and had a stem cell transplant on New Years Eve, 2008. After a three week stay in a special Multiple Myeloma ICU, I was released, put on more chemo and again tried to work as much as possible.

I retired the last day of June that year, 2009 because I was awarded 100% disability by the VA and had to end my health care and sign onto the VA system. I am happy to let you know now, that my care under the VA has been great and I have very few complaints from my ten years as a patient. As a result, I tell anyone who might need to hear, about the success I have had with the VA and can truly compare it positively to civilian hospitals because that is where I began my care. I urge all veterans to get checked out and invest the time in having yourself examined for any Agent Orange associated diseases, of which many are difficult to discern, such as MM and Ischemic heart disease. A mild update that things seem to be getting worse for treatment in the past year, as I had to wait almost three months to visit the pain clinic, a high priority 100% disabled patient.

My father being a commercial pilot and having my commercial pilots license also, I love to read the books involving all pilots. Especially the helicopter pilots who I have the utmost respect for and most likely would have also become, but for the fact I wanted to do my two years and get back to my new wife.

I get somewhat excited when I read stories in which I recognize individual names, 101st Airborne/Airmobile, Camp Evans, Camp Carroll, FB Rakkasan, Thua Thien Providence, I Corp. And battles such as Ripcord, and LamSon 719, the ARVN invasion into Laos supported by 3rd Bde, 101St AB/AM. I always have a watchful eye for friends I went through my army schooling with, or classmates from high school, or college. Those things are just little nuggets that bring more reality into my head and add a little meaning for me. I can't speak for others, but I'm sure a lot read for that familiarity or to add new and different experiences to the mix.

Another story I want to tell is that of the veterans and their lives after returning and attempting to integrate back into society. Mine is of just one type of veteran's return. That of a married man returning with no children and trying to start a new life with a wife he has spent little or no time with. From all of the reading I have done, I think this is a fairly common story as it appears that many young man and woman decided to join in wedlock prior to the serviceman leaving for training, or in my case, a few months before shipping over seas, due to a fortunate change in my Army career path.

All of these individual story lines will trend into many different paths as do the varied segments which describe the war listed earlier, but end in similar situations.

Whether married prior to training or after training, I believe the reasons were mostly akin. In our case, June and I were engaged in 1968 following her graduation and my Junior year in college. We planned to be engaged for several years while I finished college and she grew in her tenure in her job working as a unit clerk in one of the three city hospitals.

We knew we wanted children, but not soon and probably two if we could be lucky enough to be given one of each. I was majoring in education, minoring in business and had just earned my private, then my commercial pilot's license. I was also an avid painter/artist favoring flowers and seascapes and later began carving animals and selling all at local craft shows. I was not sure which direction I would go, but was leaning toward following in my Father's shoes by joining the company he had been flying for since 1955, and had plans to move in that direction, with his help.

June and I were having a great time during our dating and engagement, spending the majority of our free time together and going to the beach mostly every weekend during the summer, with her eight year old niece in tow most of the time.

She went with us on many dates and quite a few flights in my Dad's Cessna 172 Skyhawk. The previous year when I had to register for the draft, I checked in with the Army recruiter and asked about flying helicopters since I already had my fixed wing license. I was told that it was a three year enlistment and continued on my way back to college while two of my best friends joined the Air Force for a four year commitment. June and I flew mostly local and to nearby beaches when possible, usually taking her sister, niece and or her Mom.

I was working in a local hardware store around class schedules and Saturdays for the second consecutive year, as well as a job at UPS for four hours early in the morning, unloading tractor trailers. I saved enough money to get June the engagement ring we had previously picked out and we became engaged August 28, 1968. I had originally planned on graduating after nine semesters instead of eight because I started out playing football, and was taking lower credit loads in the fall semesters to carry over to the ninth semester because of the football schedule. I kept the lighter load because of my part time job after stopping football my sophomore year because of two separated shoulders and severe migraine headaches.

The following year as June turned 19, I received my draft notice, and went for my physical in Philadelphia on 7/20/69, the day of the first lunar landing. I passed with no problems and was assigned a 9/4/69 report date. Our initial thoughts were to get married after my tour was over, after 9/71. As time grew closer we started considering the possibly of getting married earlier, after one of my schools.

The problem was, I didn't know what my MOS (Military Occupational Specialty) was going to be, but it was fairly common knowledge that draftees were overwhelmingly assigned to the infantry (11B MOS), but I had four years of college, two years of ROTC, and I had my commercial pilots license. But, still, didn't have a clue as to how they chose what MOS I would be assigned after basic training.

We would have to wait. No time between basic and AIT (Advanced Infantry Training), and one week leave between AIT and Vietnam. But we were young and in love and this was a few generations ago, so we struggled with the concern of not being man and wife, with me going into a war zone and maybe never having another chance. The Government life insurance at that time was $10,000 and not even considered by us, in fact I was not even aware of that at the time. We did not discuss me not coming back outright, but obviously wanted to share that special bond, so kept the considerations open to the fates. We never even mentioned the option of going to Canada as we were both disgusted with those who chose to do so, without considering and taking other alternatives.

September fourth came very quickly. I spent most of the night with June, and went home early in the morning to say goodbye to my parents, and my brother and his family. My brother, two years my senior, but married with a child, was very upset that I was drafted, he and his wife had tried to get June and I to go ahead and get married, but we had not wanted to rush into it. My Mom drove me into the city armory and said goodbye.

All of the new inductees were standing by, waiting for the bus to take us to Philadelphia for processing and someone tapped me on the shoulder. A good family friend, one of the pilot's wives had come to tell me goodbye and wish me good luck. I loved her like a second Mom and their son was also a pilot a year older than me and in line to start training soon with Capitol, as I was hoping to be able to do. She assured me that I would be able to follow the same path as her son when I returned, but in 1971 there were major airline pilot backlogs as the war was winding down and many pilots were exiting all of the services, and I needed a job right away.

I was bused to Philadelphia, sworn in and while standing in rows, a sergeant came down the aisles tagging every other man for the Marines. We were of course all draftees and I had no idea that I could go into the marines. I didn't really have a preference other than I felt I had a better chance to get into air traffic control or flying surveillance planes, or at least something other than infantry with the Army. All I knew of the Marines was John Wayne, Aldo Ray and sand fleas at Parris Island, and that every marine was trained as an infantry soldier. I knew little more about the Army other than my uncle being in command of the Ranger training in Fort Benning, and the army had B1 bird dog Piper and Cessna spotter planes.

I was put on a train in Philadelphia with the group of selectees and rode to Fort Bragg, NC that afternoon. We were lined up just like in the movies, marched to a building where we were given a duffle bag and then went down the line being handed out gear based on your size, as judged by the person handing you that piece of equipment, no questions.

Next we went to barracks and dropped our gear and onto the shot line where both arms were pricked by needles and shot with pneumatic guns and handed your yellow injection book (I still have mine). Some guys passed out and were removed from the line as we moved to the next station which was dog tags. Name, SSN, faith, blood type. My blood type was stamped AB Positive which I found out years after I was discharged that the typing was incorrect. Lucky for me that I never was badly wounded!

Final stop, baldness. All hair disappeared in about 45 seconds. Some were really comical as they dropped their hippie or Afro hair and looked like a different person while others, myself included had only about an inch of hair to start with. Now we all looked the same convict type, minus the ID number across the chest, the first goal of the green machine.

We were marched back to the barracks and stood down until further notice. Card games and craps games broke out on almost every lower bunk and the money started flowing. Away from me! I had only brought about $30 and that was fleeced quickly because I thought Mom had schooled me well in craps, but I had obviously not been a good student with that either. She must have been taking my pennies to teach me a lesson, but poor me would have to do without anything until I could get in touch with my parents. Fortunately, I didn't need any cash until after my first pay day and I found out that the toiletries, brass cleaning supplies and shoe polish required, had to purchased, but would be deducted from our first pay.

While I was in a corner sulking about my poor gambling skills an announcement was made to fall out with our gear in full fatigue uniform and baseball cap. We were divided into companies alphabetically and many of us were to board busses to be transferred to Fort Jackson, SC. The reason for the transfer, was that we were one of the last of the draftee groups in the system before the lottery system took place, and as a result, we were in what became the largest draft calls which had swamped basic training units across the country and had to be made to fit in wherever possible. Other groups were headed for Georgia and Louisiana.

A further explanation of the overproduction of inductees can be explained by the fact that within the three months of the basic training process, all units in training cycle were called to a general assembly for an announcement.

It was explained to the massive group of young men, filling all stand only areas of the building as well as formed outside around all open exit doors so that all could hear, that the draft system was being changed from the existing selection process to a lottery system. The crowd erupted with boos and complaints as the draftees and a sizable percentage of the enlisted who did so for the option to serve four years in lieu of the draftees' two years, to choose an MOS other than infantry, thereby likely avoiding combat service in Vietnam.

To be fair, there were enlistees that did choose infantry and other MOS's with which they would probably visit Vietnam in combat rolls, for self serving or patriotic reasons. On the draftee side, there were also a percentage of young men on wayward paths who were given the choice of serving in an effort to restructure their life, or enter the penal system. Another fact that I found interesting at the time was, as described earlier, Marines that were drafted and served only two years as well. Until that point in time, having visited the Army and Air Force recruiter, but not the Marines when I signed up for the draft, I believed all Marines enlisted for three or four years. Turned out that I had no reason to boo because when the lotteries were drawn, my birthday was number was 108 which was easily in range, and incidentally for trivia, number one was 9/17. If I had made it through that last draft call, I would still have gone in a few more months.

We arrived in the wee hours of the morning without very much sleep if any. The doors quickly opened and a big, mean looking drill sergeant jumped on the bus and yelled at us to get the hell off his bus, double time.

We were to retrieve our duffel bags from the baggage compartment and line up on the lines and god help the last one. I was toward the back, but got out in a hurry only to have my bag catch on a piece of metal in the bin and tear an "L" shaped hole and spill out a few articles of clothing. I heard a loud "what the fuck do you think you are doing ass hole", as a big booted foot caught me right in the ass. I responded that my bag had gotten caught up and ripped and he got nose to nose with me, telling me that he didn't want to hear any excuses and to grab the fucking bag and shut the fuck up. I still wasn't the last one, and luckily for me, I was not assigned to his platoon.

We were divided into two companies of four platoons each and marched off to our assigned barracks realizing reveille would be sounding very soon. We actually went through the process of assigning squads, dividing to the two floors, making our bunks and storing our gear immediately, before we hit the rack. What a long day and a hard welcome to the army.

One other piece of advice my Ranger Uncle had given me about all of my training, was to try and stay somewhere in the upper middle of the trainees. Never try to excel because you get picked as a leader and have a lot of extra duties that can take a toll, don't wind up near the bottom where misery resides, and again, never volunteer.

I followed that advice through all of my training, with one exception. We were told that we cloud earn a weekend pass if we shot expert with the M16 during the third quarter of training. I saw visions of June! Basic training was like Boy Scouts and ROTC on steroids, but I was always very athletic and sort of a dare devil, but hated running long distances. We ran everywhere, luckily it was double time which isn't really a normal running pace for athletes, but the long distances did wear on me because of the equipment and heat and not being in as good of shape as I should have been.

The drill and ceremonial marching, and military drills were fun and I knew mostly everything because of ROTC. Morse code, navigating, radio techniques and weapons, all came easy as well, again because of ROTC and my flying which required use of the radio and FCC card. I really took to the

M16 and scored expert easily, even taking a smudged contact out and cleaning it in my mouth and reinserting it before one of my long range targets popped up. I didn't miss, and luckily was standing in the foxhole which allowed me the room and stance to clean it.

We weren't allowed to wear contacts, only army prescribed glasses, and the drill sergeant just shook his head while I did it. He didn't gig me because he wanted as many high scores as possible to boost the platoon and company scores which affected his performance record. I used to keep my contact case under my bunk pillow and a few days later, was gigged for my bunk not meeting regulations because I had something under the pillow that belonged in the foot locker. Of course my bunk had been tossed for effect, with my pillow left on the bed stripped and my contact lens case sitting on top of it. Nothing else was ever said, I remade my bunk, bounced a quarter off of the blanket and I still never wore my glasses, but stored my case in my foot locker.

I got the weekend pass, called the airport and reserved a flight to Washington, DC and called my Dad. The next day I was met at Dulles airport by my parents and June and the Cessna. We climbed in, Pop let me take the pilot's seat and off we went. My Mom was a white knuckle flier in the small plane, meaning she held onto straps all the way and her knuckles stayed white until we landed.

My Dad was always joking around when he flew the little plane with mild aeronautical maneuvers, dives, etc., but usually not with my Mom. He motioned to me that he was switching the fuel tanks to the tank that was showing almost empty. He said it was to check how much gas it had after it showed empty and I said I understood. The thing was however, we were just beginning to cross over one of the widest parts of the Chesapeake Bay at about 6,000 feet.

About half way over, the engine started sputtering as the tank emptied and Mom and June in the back seat started chattering concernedly and loudly, asking what was wrong. I had already switched the tank switch to the full tank before the engine quit because I wasn't interested in being in the dog house my only time with June in eight weeks. I honestly didn't want to take a chance on the plane not starting either, but I was sure I had enough altitude to glide well past the shore and already had a field in sight if needed, as we were trained. My Dad had wanted to scare them a bit more than that I think.

As a result, Dad had a rough weekend, while mine was great and we made the return flight on Sunday without Mom, but with my sister-in-law Leslie, who years later earned her private pilot license. I made it back to Columbia just before lights out. My drill sergeant asked me the next day if I had a good time and I told him yes. He then asked me if I went to Columbia and I told him no, that I flew home to Delaware. He gave me a hard look, then smiled and said it was just a local pass, but he wasn't going to say anything about it to anyone. I never knew, or asked, just assumed the pass was open, as long as I got back in 48 hours.

Much has been written and questions asked of me also, about the racial situation and the drug situation during the war. Again, that question has many answers because of all of the variables mentioned before. Primarily, your race, and whether you did drugs or not. When there and where and what MOS are probably the other major factors. I didn't see much of an issue between races, especially in the field.

There was beginning to be some segregation by choice while in the rear, with Blacks bunking together and some Hispanics bunking together, and there were some minor incidences I heard of, but remember I did not wander much, but stayed put. I've read of other severe and almost chronic situations in other units because as the war continued there became more friction, as it was at home. What I saw in the field and heard of in my units, was that everyone usually worked as a team when outside the wire, and did their own thing, within reason, inside the wire.

SECTION III: AMBUSH BY NVA

I did have one experience that tainted me for a period of time because of how it affected me personally, and I held a grudge against a black soldier for a time, finally dealing with it much later on my life by realizing that I was being unjust by placing blame on a group, rather than an individual, which was a prejudice motivated stance and very unfair and new for me and hopefully others.

I don't have any recollection of doing that prior to that incident, and have further chastised myself for distinguishing the person as black, other than for peer pressure. It could have been anyone from any race, religion of persuasion and I would have been mad, but it had nothing to do with anything but the individual, and if nothing had happened that night, it would never be mentioned.

Early in my tour, November, 1970 we were slated to make a recon into an area where a morning S2 (intelligence) air recon report detected an enemy patrol in the foothills about 25 klicks (kilometer, 1000 meters) northwest of our base. We were taking a five man team on a dusk insertion and working toward the vicinity of the siting to set up an all night observation and/or ambush, of the reported possible obscured high volume trail, to return the following morning. We usually rotated individuals based on the type of mission, short recon, long recon, cordon and security of downed helicopter, rescue mission, decoy, sniper, or backup for a unit in contact. The team was picked and a black corporal said he felt ill and didn't want to go.

He was a good guy with a good record and those things happened occasionally, but not very often because you normally took what assignments came your way, just an unwritten rule. Another friend and NCO jumped up and said that he would take the open slot, but the rest of the team said no, because he was slated to leave the following evening on his R & R to meet his wife in Hawaii, and we stood a good chance of not making it back in time for his departure. He argued that he would be OK going because it would make the wait easier for him than just sitting around, weather was to be clear and it gave us a larger priority to get back early. We agreed, but didn't like it.

The team geared up later that afternoon and had a quiet insertion after two false insertions, approximately several hundred meters from the observed site. The team picked its way quickly and covertly as possible, because of the dissipating daylight, made worse by the jungle canopy. Nearing the site, the five man team was moving approximately four to five yards apart and nearing the coordinates of the targeted trail, when an enormous explosion detonated and M16's opened up from the point and rear.

As the smoke cleared, three of the five were dead and the two survivors shaken, but alert and checking on their buddies and finding the carnage and devastation of what was considered to be a command detonated dud artillery round, probably a 155 mm, based on the destruction and debris incurred.

The point man had obviously spotted something, as his shots were seemingly simultaneous with the explosion, but was critically wounded by shrapnel, the other two KIA never had a chance, as they were closest to the blast and suffered multiple amputations while the two survivors were passing through a shallow gully in the rear, had taken light shrapnel, were temporarily deafened and mentally tasked for the short term.

They first, checked the bodies, saw that nothing could be done for their buddies, one of which was the NCO that was scheduled to meet his wife in two days. It was now pitch black, luckily one of the two radios was operational with the rear of the team and an urgent request for evacuation was made, while requesting artillery fire toward the front of the position and then around the position per H & I pre-plotted artillery targets. There was no return fire, which was very common on command detonated ambushes, as the enemy could best guarantee greater casualties by detonating as a unit was passing, rather than using a trip wire that may be detected, or might only eliminate the point man, and then they would di di mau, (get away fast), so as not to get caught by air or artillery strikes.

They positioned themselves at opposite ends of the area in an effort to establish a small perimeter for about half an hour. It was determined too dangerous to send a chopper that night as the LZ was possibly now booby trapped or not defendable by two men, and the bodies had to be guarded against any mutilation and staged for extraction.

They covered the bodies as best they could with ponchos, set up their claymores and took cover sitting back to back nearby in the brush, locked and loaded with hand grenades in their laps, pins straightened and ready for what they were sure would be an attack, while continuing harassment artillery fire through the remainder of the night and issuing situation reports. The night passed slowly without further incident, and another team was flown in and inserted at first light to rendezvous and secure the LZ for recovery of the team.

We assume that the soldier's wife most likely was already in route to Hawaii and had to be notified when she arrived, a horrible situation, and one in which we blamed the man who didn't take the mission, which I know now, was very unfair. For me personally and a few of the rest of the team, we unfortunately looked at it as a racial event and mentally blamed a group of people because of one individuals' actions. That was very unusual for me, because I had never really felt prejudice like that, but the trauma associated with this man not taking his turn, really hit me hard.

I went to school, played sports and had good friends that were black. The uncle that lived near Ft. Jackson, and his wife had retired from DC working for the government and returned to his wife's family where they bought a small diner in a very small South Carolinian town. When we traveled there as teenagers, Lee and I were shocked to see water fountains and rest rooms marked "whites only", and no blacks were allowed in the restaurant.

My uncle, having worked in DC all those years in a very integrated job, and being a Guadalcanal marine veteran, had a black friend that helped him with maintenance around the place and fed him heartily, like family, with us in the kitchen, but we were told in his presence, not to mention it to the white only customers in the dining room. What an eye opener for us in the late 50's and early 60's, and I never forgot that, including preparing June for it on her first visit, because her two best friends at work were black.

Luckily, I settled that out for me at least, about a year or so later in my life, as I started to try and reconcile some of the feelings I had related to my army life. While working at Chrysler the following year, I met and befriended several great men, two happened to be black, and took me under their wings and showed me the ropes which made it a tremendously enjoyable job for me. I owe them a lot for getting my head back on straight, at least for that social phenomenon I had enjoined. Many more issues were harbored deep in my head, hopefully to sort out as time wore on.

There were situations in training in the states where minority groups would save large spaces in chow lines for their friends who would all be signaled at the right time and that caused some angst, but was usually dealt with by nearby cadre. I know there are some very bad examples and even fraggings on record, but probably no worse than in civilian life, minus the fraggings. There were probably more arguments over music than other issues. Motown, versus country, versus rock & roll, and I liked all three, but whoever had the radio or tape player usually set the tunes, or allowed others to take turns. Just like getting a care package from home. In the field, you might get the personal items, but you shared everything edible with your buddies. If you were in base camp, you might squirrel your favorites away in a locker and share the rest, but you always shared.

While talking about the music being played, I want to mention my memories of the songs of the time and how they affected me then, and even until this day. Just as the sound of helicopters are an instant recall and sometimes anxiety for many Vietnam Veterans, also were the very popular songs of those years.

When I hear them, and I do listen to the 60's and 70's music more than all others combined, I go right back to that time in my life in my mind. "Summer in the City", by

The Loving Spoonful, takes me to the summers at the beach with June when we first started dating, a very personal one. "War", by Edwin Starr, "We Gotta' Get Out of This Place", "Don't Let Me Be Misunderstood", "House of the Rising Sun", and "Bury My Body", by The Animals were constantly played over the AFSN (Armed Forces Service Network) out in the field when secure and in all fire bases and base camps. "Paint It Black", "Satisfaction", "You Can't Always Get What You Want", "Get Off My Cloud", "Gimme Shelter", by The Rolling Stones, all drift through my mind when I reach back to my time in country. I was introduced to country music with "Okie from Muskogee", by Merle Haggard and "Crystal Chandelier", by Charlie Pride music by hooch mates. "Sitting on the Dock of the Bay", Otis Redding and others from earlier concerts where I provided security. "The Thrill is Gone", by B.B. King, "Get Together", by the Youngbloods, "What's going On", by Marvin Gaye, 'Whiter Shade of Pale, by Procol Harum, "Let It Be", "Revolution", by The Beatles and lots more, all June's and my memories. "A Hard Rain's A Gonna Fall" , "Mr.. Tambourine Man", by Bob Dylan, and way too many to mention, allow me to go back and remember key times in my life. And probably the most played song, used as a finale in just about every USO show throughout the country, "Green Green Grass of Home", which usually brought tears and sings along from the homesick and lonesome GI's.

As with many of the statistics, some dramatic incidents muddied the entire picture on race, drugs, morale and egregious behavior. They were mostly, in my opinion, less overwhelming than depicted, as negative situations usually got more attention in other areas. I do believe that what was happening in the states was driving the racial issue in Vietnam more so than visa versa.

During the war, the black KIA ratio 12.5% (5,711) as the average military aged population of 13.5% in the states during that period. The total black that served represented 10.6% (275,000). Hispanics were included in Caucasian served, but total KIA 5.2% (3070), and other races combined at 1.1%. While the total of black served was almost 3% less than the general population at the time, the KIA rate was 2% higher than than those served, so tragically, they had a higher rate of KIA. It is also more likely that the ratios were skewed the other way in the earlier years of the war, as these are the average.

As drugs go, basically you drank or did mostly drugs, drank and drugs, mostly beer and marijuana, or, maybe, did neither, but most wouldn't pass up beer or a hard drink for 10 or 25 cents respectively
. What else was there? The beer was almost always hot and stale as it sat around forever on pallets in the sun. The cans were steel, not aluminum and sometimes rusted and no pop tabs yet, but on larger bases, you could go to clubs for cold drinks. Everyone had their church key with their P38 GI can opener, on a key chain to open beer and C rations hanging from their belt loop, dog tags or D ring ready for the occasion, which I still have in my medal box. Soft drinks were as available as beer but were also hot and stale, but CocaCola could be bought in bottles and iced down from local vendors at times outside the wire or also in bases with clubs.

Some wonderful NCO's in charge in the rear would occasionally provide iced down beer and sodas on logistic runs to the field units. If I remember, the cans were 10 cents or about $1.50 for a case, and I don't remember anyone buying a case of Coke, but most of us would buy a case of beer and share. I was not around drugs very much, but they were certainly used. In fact my first night in my unit I stayed in the orderly room with two other soldiers, one coming in as I was and one leaving for the WORLD. I was dead tired and trying to get to sleep on an army cot and the other two lit up a marijuana cigarette and offered me a hit. I declined, but finally found out what marijuana smelled like and never forgot it. I never smoked, not even in Nam and usually traded my cigarettes from the hospitality packs and C rations for the meals I preferred, or gave them away, as most guys didn't want to give me what I wanted. I was very picky, especially with C's because I couldn't tolerate many of them.

There were many warnings, especially as you became a short timer of drug use and many rumors that if testing positive while out processing (tested as leaving country and leaving Ft. Lewis) or caught with anything on you, that you would not be discharged or reassigned until you were weaned off. There were stations along the way in both countries where you were encouraged to discard any contraband or items that might get you in trouble, and allowed to discard anonymously as cadre turned around and did not look. You could also be withheld if you had a severe case of VD and tales of relocation to isolated leprocy type compounds. Again, one of four Vietnam Veterans were diagnosed with VD while in country. The drugs, VD and contraband were the things that self control would reward you for, and barring being a casualty, gave you a quick shot to get home, while processing out.

Like with the other conversation points, there were certainly bad times and areas for drugs and reached almost epidemic proportions as the war continued, but not necessarily within the combat units. There were a lot of guys like me, that didn't want to be with anyone using a hard drug with them in the field, and didn't tolerate it outside of camp. Everything imaginable was available on the black market, drugs especially, but the combat units were more forward positioned and away from the big cities and major supply areas. We couldn't even get beer at times, hardly never any steaks, and had limited access to even a PX, until rotated back to a rear area or an in country R & R of a few days, which many, including me, never had, and probably would not have taken.

The other questions and concerns of people is centered around morale and degrading conduct. Morale was all over the place depending on conditions, how cherry or short you were and what you heard from home. Obviously, your morale sucked if you were in the monsoons, whether you were in the field or in the rear, because there was nowhere that the wet, wind and cold did not penetrate. What was happening in your AO could also dictate ups and downs in your daily life.

But the overall morale had much to do with what you knew from back in the World. New arrivals, radios, letters, newspapers from home and in country Stars and Stripes Armed Forces Newspaper circulations were the main source of home news and the bad things, such as Bobby Kennedy and Martin Luther King's assassinations, Kent University shootings, marches and riots had the type of effects you would imagine, and would somewhat reflect conditions in the World. While the moon landing, reports of downsizing, World Series, Super Bowl, bowl games, etc. had positive impacts on the troops, at least short term.

But whether new or short timer, you could go from 1 to 10 and back again over and over, and in short periods of time, and a lot of that was controlled by those old sweetheart letters on mail call day. Some guys received almost no correspondence and it was pitiful enough that others might share theirs to read, which could make it worse. Others would ask friends or sisters to write a buddy in need of friendship and communication. Some received letters from church groups and even school children and community groups providing care packages and letters. I received letters from elementary school children and women from church, thanks to the community, and had several corresponding back and forth letters, which I responded to, and thanked, even passed names of soldiers in need of correspondence. I truly lived for mail call and the much needed scent of June's perfume, which ironically, was "Ambush" by Dana.

I don't consider morale to be necessarily related to patriotism, and I hate to say that patriotism was almost nonexistent, in the way I discerned patriotism at the time. Remember, almost one third overall who served at my time were drafted, but that number was quite a bit higher as the war continued, than the overall average of 26%, because less were enlisting because of national sentiment and as described, the draft calls were increasing with time to the point of basic training space saturation. Draftees also comprised 32% of combat deaths. Also as the draftees increased in time and volume, were a larger percent of combat soldiers and the education level and age was likewise increasing.

Most of my basic training company had two to four years of college and were 20 to 25 years old, in fact the average age of KIA's for the entire war was 22.8 years, not much younger as commonly thought. Also, almost 80% of the enlisted had high school degrees and even higher with draftees, again skewed higher as time continues, compared to only 65% of non-military aged male Vietnam veterans and 45% in WWII.

In fact, after my drill sergeant read off my name for Advanced Infantry School, I requested to see the Captain to ask why the infantry, when I had college and pilots license. He simply told me that contrary to belief, the infantry needed smarts more than any other MOS, because in order to survive you had to have intelligence. He further explained the composition of our company and indicated that the few that were not well educated would be cooks and clerks in many circumstances, because they had certain requirements to meet for the infantry training and Vietnam.

Many of the common myths portrayed of Vietnam veterans are not true and resulted in many derogatory concepts formed during the era. I will enclose a study from VVof.org compiled which include these and other fictions and exaggerations which were misconstrued to portray certain points to be made. Many of these resulted, in my opinion, in some of the pessimistic views the citizenry had of returning veterans and were based on highly exaggerated and or over publicized information. Heck, I wouldn't even hire ME, if I allowed myself to believe some of those pigeon holes we were put into, and I'm always for the underdog. It's the mob mentality and it makes people with reason disregard their good sense, but maybe a lot of them didn't have the common sense they were born with.

Fourteen years after I came home, they decided to put on the ticker tape parade for Vietnam veterans in New York City. I wasn't impressed, didn't even look at it on TV or read about it until much later, and would not even consider going to participate, but not because I was upset for not getting any recognition. I thought it was too little too late, and parades aren't even feasible when the country is rotating troops in and out to whatever units needs the manpower.

How could you ever assimilate people for a parade until the fighting was over, but 10 years after Vietnam was won by the North, and 10 years after the last two American Marines died of a rocket attack the day before the NVA overran Saigon and chased us all out? Not to mention that we didn't win, why have a parade if we let the enemy win? Many of us had already visited their local VFW Lodges shortly after returning, to find that they really didn't want us there, as our war, wasn't really a WAR, but a police action, and was lost! Oh, we were welcome to join and drink at the bar with them, but they didn't really want us to lay any war stories on them, because they wouldn't compare with theirs. Little did they know, that most of us probably wouldn't have done that any way, which they would, if they remembered their celebrated returns home. I went through that myself, drank one beer, alone, walked out and never returned. Now I'm getting requests from them and other veteran organizations every year, which I just throw away. I guess they need members, and money now that their core is evaporating.

I think a lot of Vietnam veterans felt relief from the parade, I didn't, but I'm glad if anyone was able to get some closure, however, it probably didn't put a stop to anyone's PTSD, or bring a marriage back together again, or cure someone of drug addiction, because PTSD had only started being recognized and treated in full about 6 years before the parade. And why have General Westmoreland lead the parade? John McCain and the other prisoners should have led the parade, even though they had already had one, and were apparently upset they were given a parade when every other returnee got shamed. They deserved it as well as all of the severely wounded and their families as well as those families of the killed and missing.

When I speak of patriotism during the war, I am not saying that I am not, or we were not patriotic people. We mostly were and are now, but at the time, we didn't agree with, nor did we understand fully, why we were there, nor how the war was being conducted. Remember, we were younger but better educated than our fathers and grandfathers in WWI and WWII, respectively and in general. Our fathers being older, as the war in Europe had been going on a few years before we joined with the attack on

Pearl Harbor in 1941 and it was a world war and the draft had an older base to start with. With the advanced technology, we were more educated in what we were getting into than our predecessors, which made us more knowledgeable of what was likely to happen to us.

I am again, speaking as serving toward the end of the crisis as it was winding down and demonstrations were rampant as we walked through airports on our way there and anywhere we traveled. I'm sure that earlier on during the war there was a lot of rah-rah, but not when I was there, however, that doesn't mean that I would not do it all over again and I'm not proud. I am proud that I served, would do it again without thinking about it and encouraged my son to serve after he tried college for a short time, needing to obtain more structure in his life. Growing up with grandfathers and fathers and uncles fighting in the two big wars, and Korea, how can you not be at least somewhat patriotic?

It was a war that was fought like no other, as discussed, and there began to develop an unrest not seen in such abundance before. My uncle, a true lifer, chose to retire instead of going back for a second tour. I asked my aunt prior to her passing a few years ago, why he made that choice and she told me that he didn't like the disrespect that was developing between lower to higher ranks as well as the increased drug situation. As the war progressed, so did the misconduct toward rank as well as fraggings, dramatically worse in some units than others. He was a soldier, an officer that always demanded respect as he demanded it from his children and nephews. He was a solid officer and held an exemplary record and I've read books of his unit noting respect for him, but he had enough, and came back a little meaner, bidding his dream of becoming a General, with having to leave his family again, goodbye Vietnam, goodbye army.

My patriotism for the war was low, but for our country, it never wavered. I have always been patriotic even having been drafted, I got goose bumps marching and drilling to the military patriotic music as the band played and you stepped down with your left foot on the base drum beat, especially during ceremonies. Sure I resented what was happening at home and the total disrespect that was shown by the populace toward anyone in uniform, but especially the name calling and false assertions. I was told the war was to keep communism from spreading, but lost sight of that as time wore on while in country. Wasn't it unpatriotic to those of us that either joined or accepted our responsibility when drafted, to disrespect us? Not the demonstration, but the ridicule, the name calling, and the draft card and flag burnings. That sure sounds like lack of patriotism to me. I also began to get really pissed about the false information that flowed through the airwaves. Everyone that was in the field knows incidents of false documentation of records for earning awards took place, suffered somehow because of the black market, or saw the rules broken for special self improving advantages.

Sure there were atrocities, show me one war before or after in which there weren't any. Many atrocities are never reported or dumbed down so as not to offend the masses. Yes, My Lai was horrible and a total annihilation of that village by some heartless and evil soldiers, but it is worse, because it was ordered, and most likely to Calley, not by Calley, and held back from even being reported for a long time. But there were real heroes there as well, the pilots that put themselves between villagers and the shooters to stop it, and those who didn't participate, of which little was told, and those who reported it. I happened to be going through my training in FT. Benning months before the trial, while the preparation and hype for the Calley trial was beginning, followed it closely when possible, and could not believe, that with all of the evidence and first hand testimony, he was charged and sentenced, but never served jail time. He was sentenced to life imprisonment subject to hard labor at Ft. Leavenworth, Kansas, but kept in quarters while the charges were dismissed for three and half years, having never served any jail time. Why? It was suggested that his troops had considered him for a fragging, but never carried it out obviously, for unknown reasons. Possibly because the brass knew it came from much higher than him and they took it easy on their scapegoat.

Sometimes, bad acts are done with partial or full consciousness and other times they are a result of fright or reaction to stimulus, but they continue to happen. None of us know what we will truly do, until we have to deal with it, and hopefully most people won't get that chance. It's not just choices in war, where life and death are concerned, that your adrenaline goes crazy. Often your mind moves your body too fast or, or it may make you slow down and cower and anything in between. If lucky, your conscience should help you avert participation, which again, I feel is part of common sense.

We would all like to think we would do the right thing when circumstances call for it, but anyone who has been in a fight of any type, including dealing with a life threatening disease, doesn't know until the time is there, and many of us who have been there have seen many different reactions from different types of people, ourselves included. Some that surprise us in many ways and some that were probably expected. There can even be multiple reactions by the same people, after all, that's all we are is people, human beings, reacting genetically to stimulus, fight or flight and maybe differently at different times, because our mind and body are reacting differently.

Sometimes offenders of harsh acts are punished and sometimes they are not. We in the public will never know everything, and most likely not even all who participated and especially how devastating they are. As in the statistical war and the reasons of war, information is sometimes altered, added, or redacted, all to the will of the authorities and how deep they feel the story goes, or how much grief it will cause will determine how it is controlled.

From degrading and defacing bodies, one of the most common and may become a fad, such as collecting ears among soldiers, to torturing prisoners and throwing them out of helicopters to make their buddy talk, to murdering innocent civilians, to building false hero's and heroins to build up war support, giving out full scholarships and denying the event as reported much later. To totally discounting facts and decoy stories, until truth resounds because the false stories escape to families, to incidents where families aren't even told about friendly fire deaths of professional athlete/soldiers. To not being able to view remains because it doesn't match the story, or even friendly fire incidents in general, not always reported, most, not reported at all. Whatever those reasons are, I feel that the truth is what is really needed. Let us decide for ourselves, with our beliefs and conscience, what result it will have on us, don't try to decide for us, let the reactions be what they are.

There is too much untruth and misinformation and seems to come from the highest sources, which opens the doors for those at lower levels to do the same thing, without fear of retribution. The truth has to come from the top, otherwise there will be little our no belief that there is truth anywhere. And without truth, how can there ever be credibility. Ask anyone who knows me well enough to vent in front of them, if I don't always question government information, especially concerning war and politics, but why would a common sense person just stop there?

Questioning keeps my mind working and keeps me looking and hoping that I may someday expect the truth. I know that I'll never see it on a steady and regular basis, if at all, but there are very reliable news gatherers that provide the truth, as common sense and honorable people, so you have to come to the real results yourself, using your common sense evaluating the "truthful" data. It should not be any other way anywhere, especially in our country, and that truth, is what any patriot should not only want, but demand, anything else belongs where dictators rule and puppets serve and live, and live to serve.

I guess patriotism was somewhat personalized for us over there, at least for me. I had very patriotic heroes in Vietnam, a Captain that refused an order to try to retake a hill after two costly attempts, in equipment and blood. He volunteered to go it alone but would not order any of his remaining soldiers to follow. Of course they all would have gone, because they were all patriotic, and loyal to him, and would not let their leader go alone, but patriotic for their immediate team and unit, not the war and who ran it. The order was receded and he was later, softly removed from his command, but became a sort of folk hero and widely respected. He continued with the brigade in an assistant staff position where I worked with him and was a legend to the entire division, at least to the non coms and below, and continues to be held in that high regard as a brave patriot by those who know and served with him, a real hero.

Or the very patriotic OH-6 Loach pilot who flew on pink and white teams, but more often went aloft alone when no one else would fly, no matter what the situation or danger, or how bleak the weather, he would find a way. He used that little bird to remove WIA, KIA, make one man assaults, ammo, food and water resupply runs, into and out of holes in the jungle that seemed impossible to even see the ground below, let alone navigate through. He was amazing, a hero, as were many, many others.

Everyone over there was a hero or heroine and a patriot, that I encountered at work, especially as loosely defined in current times, but more certainly as defined then and I loved that we were Americans, but did not feel "patriotic or non patriotic" in the way people get so irritated about an athlete kneeling, to draw attention to a very tragic problem happening within the country that is just a small part of the larger race relation issues going on.

I'm patriotic, I stand for the flag, but Not because I have to, and I certainly do not feel like those athletes are disrespecting the flag when it is their right to protest a problem of that magnitude, especially when they do a hundred times more than the rest of us do individually in their communities to help the less fortunate, no matter what color their skin, or their religion. Yes, they can afford to help them because they excelled in their field, the way we would all like to excel.

Just listen, they very much respect the Armed Forces and the jobs they do, and in no way disrespect them or the flag. I don't get all hyper and ballistic if someone doesn't stand, and rant that I fought, to give them the privilege to stand. That's not why I was there, I was there because it was the patriotic response bred into me, I was there because I was chosen to go, I certainly didn't go to Vietnam in order that someone HAS TO stand, or has to do anything, but so that they CAN stand and CAN constitutionally do anything they want in our democratic country, as long as law abiding citizens.

I don't want people to disrespect the flag/country, and I don't think those people kneeling are showing any disrespect toward the country or the Armed Forces at all, but respect for trying to make things equal for everyone. They don't exhibit disrespect. The people slouching next to you drinking a beer or eating a hotdog or pretzel, with a hat on their head, holding their camera to their face, laughing and talking, acting like they are singing while pretending to know the words, are the ones disrespecting the flag. One vulgar response from one who "pretends" to have moral authority, but has absolutely zero, and people get real "patriotic", under false pretenses as far as I'm concerned.

Kneeling, sitting or standing while reflecting and being quiet is good enough for me. To my thinking, making a lame argument like that, is a type of accelerationism, a political social theory, that capitalism should be expanded or sped up to bring radical social change. Change needed for the further separation of races, by antagonizing groups which bolster the opposing extremist, in an attempt to deter the different races, religions or other social groups. Very similar to the Russian attack of our elections on social media recently.

We can't afford, in my opinion, as a nation to go backwards in history or recreate those serious mistakes of the past, we can only work towards ending the divisive rhetoric and unite as one nation, and then work on uniting all nations. In retrospect, this is what I hoped to gain by going to Vietnam, to prevent the spread of communism, which is what we were told, by getting far as possible from a dictatorship such as we were fighting with the help of the Chinese and Russians, to move forward into the future so my grandkids can have an honest chance to enjoy their children and their future children, and so on.

How many Vietnam veterans truly and honestly felt good and proud about the government when you were there? All I ever heard was cursing and complaining about almost everything connected to who sent us there and why. Be honest, because I didn't see the positive attitudes. I saw peace jewelry everywhere even on steel pots and necklaces, just like at home. Our favorite salute was the middle finger (still my personal favorite) or peace sign, not to the flag, and not to your superior officers. You wore a disgruntled, scared frown most of the time I saw you, or looked in a mirror. Did you salute the flag unless at a KIA ceremony, or a big wig medal ceremony?

I heard loud music everywhere on encampments and don't ever remember retreat or reveille being played wherever I was. No one would have stopped what they were doing anyway. I don't ever remember saluting at all while in country, not even to an officer in the rear, maybe I did, because I did respect a lot of officers, but not all, and maybe because they didn't expect it from us.

Standing for a song is not necessarily respect for the flag, telling the truth and being honest and respectful to EVERYONE, is patriotic and expected, especially in America. Demand the truth if you are patriotic! I know all of those things made us resentful to government and the forces in our society that were causing all of the marches and demonstrations. Remember the comments to short timers, by FNG's when asking about how they would act and what they were going to do in celebration, when getting back to the world, telling them that they would be hard-pressed to do them because of the temperature of the public. Did the draft dodgers act patriotic, because I sure don't see it that way, and we have had a few as presidents. Canada reports 20,000 to 30,000 young men defected there, while the BBC claims up to 60,000 in all fled the US, including deserters, approximating the number of dead young men and women killed during the war. Is that a patriotic trade, along with flag and draft card burnings?

But somewhere along the line, the exact point I can't remember, but near 1985, the tide started to change, and the public started taking on a different concept of us, even started showing some respect. Was it the ticker tape parade, the new war movies, or more probably the Vietnam veterans and their loved ones, changing those older concepts with their actions, and not the wrongly predicted or mis-portrayed actions expressed and expected?

Maybe that is what led to the social network phenomenon I mentioned earlier, of new mutual love and respect for the Vietnam veteran, if not just heaped on us by ourselves and our loved ones. I am not totally sure which is correct, but I stay away from it for the most part, save it for the younger, current and returning veterans, and hope toward the future that we continue to do the right thing for the new veterans, as a committed, honest populace.

Patriots, heroes? How about the nurses the pilots and crewmen, the artillery units, the mechanized units, all of the non-combat support units, navy ships, navy patrol boats, aircrews, etc. It took everyone there for you to make it back alive. I would have helped any service person I saw if needed, still will, but not because of the flag, because of the person. I didn't want a parade. I don't know anyone that did, because this was a different kind of war. Most of us, excluding Marine units, went over as individuals, fought or served with a unit of individuals, and came back home as individuals, but also, part of a whole group of service members who served our tour of up to 13 months for the marines.

Many of us DEROS'd when we came back home, got out early, we were finished with active service, we didn't want a parade, we didn't care about medals, we weren't career soldiers, but we did not expect to be treated like freaks simply because we WERE patriotic and went, when we could have gone to Canada, or deserted, with the hope of being treated as positive additions to society when we were allowed to come back, without penalty. They couldn't have been any more scared to go to war than I was, I'm sure. My common sense and my heart aches, when I rethink this process. January, 1977 was too soon to throw that one in our face, never, was all that was acceptable to me at the time.

As mentioned earlier in this writing, I believe each war is worse on the soldier as we go backwards in time.

Our fathers and grandfathers were away from home for the duration, often without leave, for years. They suffered in ways we cant imagine because of the technology of war regressing in sync with retracing history. The positive point in this entire conversation is the shrinkage in human losses of the warriors as we go forward and we should all hope and do what we can to keep that trend improving, and hopefully we continue to learn from our mistakes and do move forward.

I know that it seems that those people that participated in those demonstrations, or just agreed with those who did were mostly only mad at the authorities, as I feel somewhat ill now, sending our young toward battle today, when I believe there are better options. June and I sure didn't like Chris or his friends going, but we supported them, even after June had said many times after I came home, that she would never let a son of her's go to war. Even though we didn't agree with the wisdom of the entire scenario, we kept those feelings private, born of experience and support of him and them and us.

The difference is that I don't take it out on anyone, I just grumble to myself until writing this story, and since June is no longer with me, I know she would agree with me still. I don't hold anyone personally accountable for those demonstrations of hate and malice, it was more of a mob mentality which usually isn't good for anyone, but gives a false courage for the participants.

Chris and one of his friends came to me before they were deployed, both unsure and scared of what they might encounter. Chris actually waited until he was almost there via letter, I responded immediately with the longest, most sensitive letter I had ever written him, and I did write often.

During basic training he wrote that he was concerned that his nephews Kyle and Kam would not remember him, as he was smelling the honeysuckle at Parris Island and feeling homesick. I assured him that no one would forget him, but only respect him, especially those two little guys who looked to him like a big brother and mentor. His friend came over before he left for his deployment and wasn't directly headed toward danger, but as every Marine does, guessed he probably would, and maybe, wished he might. I gave them both the same advice my uncle had given to me and I had given to those three soldiers over thirty years earlier.

Keep your head down, remember what you were taught, listen to your superiors and those who have been there, and don't do anything stupid, and you'll be fine. Just come back. I never heard from Chris about that letter, if it might have helped him, so I asked when we picked him up when his ship docked with Kyle and Kam in tow, and he said that it had gotten lost for months and he had just received it on his was back, so it wasn't able to provide any comfort to him.

That reminds me of my receiving a care package in March, 1971 a little late for my 24th birthday, while I was near the DMZ at Camp Carrol, a small firebase north east of Khe Sanh, during Lam Son 719 ARVN invasion of Laos. I settled in on top of my bunker to open it up, only to find an errant Christmas package from home, including cassette tapes from my parents and June. June had sent me a new song by the Carpenters, just for me, of "Merry Christmas Darling" and a bunch of cookies, vienna sausages, sugar free cool aid for our canteens, etc. She had also wondered why I had not ever mentioned the gifts in my letters home prior to my thank you letter back. Of course I shared my package, but kept the tapes and listened to them time and again, especially the song, which is one of my most favorite Christmas songs still today.

That operation was the assignment that I had volunteered for when my first sergeant came to me and explained that there was a very large operation coming up and it was top secret, and I could not talk about it. I had not been seriously wounded and had less combat than the others I was working with, and he wanted to see if I would go rather than the totally new or those who had suffered from serious wounds. He would have us draw straws if I chose not to volunteer, but I agreed to go, not knowing anything about what I was going to do other than become a forward radio relay for the operation, for no reason than to be fair. Camp Carrol was the firebase I would be operating from, for the approximately two to three months in support of the Laos invasion. I flew there via helicopter toward the end of January and came back a day before I left on R & R in early April. I'm not sure if I went back there or not after R & R as I just can't seem to remember much detail of the entire deployment, or after, with the exception of my wonderful R & R with June.

AMBUSH

BOOK III: HALLUCINATIONS

SECTION IV: AMBUSH BY HALLUCINATION

FIRST HOSPITAL ADMISSION, 12/31/12 (Four months after June's passing)

I started several months earlier, at Physicians and friends suggestion, seeing a VA Psychologist and Counselor. Already on the drug fluoxetine as a prophylactic for migraines as part of my original medication for my diagnosis of Multiple Myeloma (light chain deposition disease) and stage IV kidney disease. My Psychologist increased by two the fluoxetine medication to aide in my deepening depression, with instructions to increase by one or two if depression worsened.

I was suffering through the holidays with a bronchial problem, began running a mild fever and asked my son to take me into the VA emergency room per my Oncologist. I was admitted after examination and assigned a bed in a waiting area until a room was ready. While waiting for a bed the old series "Twilight Zone" was playing on the TV and I can still remember two of the episodes I watched while laying there and wonder if that had some effect on the mind games that were beginning with me. I was kept over night and told my son had been called to come and get me on New Years Day.

There weren't many staff members working on the holiday and I couldn't get anyone to confirm what time he was coming. The longer I sat in the bed the more disoriented I became. I started getting up and wondering out of the room and a nurse came in asking me questions to which I apparently couldn't answer to her satisfaction and, after conferring with others, she said I was going to have to stay longer and they would notify my son. Once in the room I began having hallucinations (a common occurrence during childhood while running a fever) and thought a man was trying to stick me with a needle while in bed. The room and hospital seemed totally different to me than the VA hospital I was accustomed to. I thought it was now in the city by a hotel and my ward, in a basement area which afforded the man easy entry, while actually on the fourth floor where the inpatient ward was located. The only familiar thing to me was a nurse who worked part time in the Chemo Ward but was also working on my floor that day. I complained to the other nurses and asked to be put in a different room as I was under the impression this man had found a way to stick me with a needle through the adjacent wall. They and another patient assured me that that was not possible but I left my room and went to the nursing station to find Tiffany, the nurse I was familiar with. I pleaded with Tiffany because of our relationship through my chemo to move, me pleading with her to reason with me about knowing each other and how she knew I couldn't make this up, but they were not able to accommodate me.

I was visited by the head of the Psychiatry Department of the hospital who reviewed my recent history and decided to put me on an additional, more powerful psychiatric drug to evaluate my progress. I slept for quite a while vividly dreaming the entire time that in an adjacent room, other nurses, male and female were competing in some wild video game to achieve special classifications at work. I was invited to try my hand at it and while doing so, bettered all of their scores which they attributed to the drugs I was on. My hallucinations continued to grow and get more vivid until I saw no reality at all, as I felt like I was in a dream world with no control and no way out.

Over the next day or so my Oncologist visited me and got me somewhat calmed down. It was determined to take me off of the new drug and as my fever subsided I began to return to normal with the exception of thinking my kids had forgotten about me and I felt that they had brought my dog which was wondering in and out of the hospital with someone I didn't know. My primary worry was always how Maggie was faring in my absence and I had absolutely no control of her. That person was also creating difficulties for me to the extent I couldn't be trusted to be discharged.

Each subsequent visits of my Nephrologist and Disease Control specialists proved confusing to me. I do have memories, but they are overly exaggerated in their content, as my mind spiced them up substantially by bringing my kids and their spouses into the mix. They were involved with the doctors and a few of the nurses in a real estate deal selling their homes, which I thought was extremely detrimental to all of them and me because my daughter's house was in my name. I was only in the hospital for 4 or 5 days but it felt much longer to me. My Oncologist is the one who arranged for my discharge and the orders to resume my normal activities and medications at home., sans the new psychotic drug and only the fluoxetine for my depression.

SECOND HOSPITAL ADMISSION, 7/3/14

Approximately one week prior to the second admission on July 3, 2014 I began having hallucination episodes at home while again running a fever. Several days before I was taken to the hospital I began having strange episodes of people visiting me in bed explaining that my wife wasn't really dead. The initial visits of these people were three sisters and friends of the family that my daughter had grown up with. They were all sitting in and around the bed excited that they had found the information which they were told that claimed she wasn't really dead and the coroner determined that she had lost some of her memory and was working with her in some secluded location.

As the night wore on I ended in a strange place where a carnival like entourage celebrated the occasion. Costumes, lots of people some of whom I knew and some disguised, and a festive atmosphere, but secretive at the same time. Most family and friends were also there. Colored lights loud music, lots of celebrating and even some sort of carnival rides. Next thing I knew I was back in my room and the same thing was going on there but to a much smaller extent and the intent turned from friendly consoling and celebrating, to strange demands to provide the return of my wife.

I began becoming provoked and pushed around and the people were there one minute and gone the next. I thought they were trying to provoke me in some way and made up my mind to find them in the total dark, as I was becoming extremely agitated. I grabbed my big Bowie knife and started searching for them. Caught one and put the knife to his throat and told him to stay put and tell the others to come out of hiding. They would not, so I grabbed my gun and told them I was going to find them and scare them out of my house. I couldn't corner them but thought they were hiding in a closet in bathroom so I placed the large revolver against the wall in my bedroom and angled it to fire through the walls. Not to hit anyone but to scare them.

Next I thought they were in the crawl space and placed a smaller 22 caliber gun above the baseboard to fire through the walls just above the floor, and finally when I thought, they were leaving I placed the gun by the window molding and angled it to fire into the woods behind the house. Maggie, my dog was barking like crazy and chasing me around while I was going through these antics. I believe, the time frame, from the knife through the three shots lasted less than five minutes, but really have no idea how fast or slow it was.

I must have fallen to sleep after that and my room was a mess. I let my daughter know I had discharged the guns the next day when we talked, and my son came over and took all my guns and big knives to his house. The only damage I did other than holes in walls was damage to my new shower I had just recently installed, the bullet smashing the glass on the control panel wall.

During the next few days my kids and older grandsons kept visiting me and bringing meals, but I didn't eat much and continued to take my medications including morphine for the cancer pain. Things got worse for me mentally. I went through many different episodes with people and voices visiting me and asking me to do unusual things. It started the next night with voices when I thought I was witnessing a trio of ladies acting as fortune tellers sitting at my dining room table while I was sitting in my chair in the adjoining sunroom. There was a flower painted ceramic pig (one of my wife's collection) sitting on the table that I thought was the cute, painted face of one of the women, who I thought was a dead ringer to Snow White two years later.

At one point I thought the three sisters were at the table listening also, and my two granddaughters were running around playing hide and seek. The tellers were playing some kind of game with me about my past and future and were using supposedly expensive minerals/jewels as rewards when I was correct about answers, but the game was to gain control of me totally, by bringing up things from my past and predicting shortfalls for my future. As the game progressed and I accumulated some prizes, I was constantly being penalized by bringing fabrications from our past and even introducing a local police officer that was part of the group and was threatening to arrest me for discharging the guns the night before. Turned out that he was an old acquaintance of mine when I lived in Dover from 3rd to 6th grade, never liked me, followed my career in sports and business along with others in the group and had developed a grudge against me over the years. I was shown videos where he had actually impersonated me doing bad things in order to convince me and others that the videos were me.

As time wore on, various characters began to develop and join with the ones already identified. One voice in particular and disguised as my neighbor and landscape vendor, began to appear to be the leader of the group. Up to a dozen more began integrating into the conversation until it was nonstop talking back and forth. I was actually responding verbally in the beginning and subliminally if someone was with me or I didn't want them to hear me....but they always knew what I was thinking and feeling.

I called and got no answer and even walked to my neighbor's house that night and asked why he was doing this to me. He obviously denied it and tried to settle me down and then called my son Chris (takes care of his lawn also) and told him he was worried about me because of what I was saying to him. Chris came over to check on me and I confided to him that it was really happening, not just in my head. The voices also helped me remember a girl I had been nice to and given a little kiss on the cheek in 6th grade because others were making fun of her. She was one of the three fortune tellers at the table, and of course she told me about this and asked if I remembered it, so I said that I did, but I really did not. She stood up for me throughout the ordeal and appeared in the regression two years later.

Other people who knew myself or June over the years came in and out of these two sessions, two years apart and most became progressively more confusing and condemning to me, but some offered comfort and compassion at extreme times to keep me going when I started losing it. As the fortune telling session continued I was totally focused on one dressed as a gypsy and not the other two nor the other voices of which there were more than six at the time.

I began staring into her eyes from across the rooms until I rattled her. She tried not to look at me as they continued to rip into my past but when she did, I locked her there. She had to try and ask for help subliminally without moving her lips and the others subliminally told her not to look at me, but she couldn't keep it up. I started picking their game apart by stating I knew where they had cameras located and that I knew how they were controlling my phones TV and computer. I also told them I knew how they controlled the caf doors by adding mechanisms into the hinges to control them and knew they had put a lifting mechanism on the table to control it, even cut a trap door in the floor to the crawl space, rigged windows and attic in order to gain quick and unseen entry and exit of the house.

That is when they brought the cop into it complete with lights flashing outside. We bartered back and forth as the game went on until I thought I had the upper hand with how they were controlling me. I began to collect the majority of the rewards and they started backing off a little like I was starting to get out from under their control, until another controlling voice told them that I had no control and it all changed back with me on the defensive. They had put implants in my eyes, head, etc., with cameras and speakers all over the house, so that I had no place of privacy. They could even feel pain when I encountered it, knew when someone was entering the driveway, and told me how I was to try and get rid of them so we could continue. This went on for several days and nights without me going to bed. I was found in all sorts of unexplainable situations when family came in.

It finally came down to one person supposedly controlling everything, with me not really understanding why. More than a dozen were involved and I was discerning more and more as time wore on. They would not let me take medicine, had a doctor with them (one of the ones who said they had control of June). Found many ways to keep me awake including telling me that I had to practice slogans on the telephone pretending to be a black football star of the same name moving from college to professional and involved with their scheme. I had to change my accent and do radio ads over and over and even call prospective accounts and pretend to be asking for contributions for promoting their products, ironically connected to my retired profession.

As time wore on I uncovered the identity of a contractor I had exposed legally years ago for illegal discarding contaminated material and misrepresenting real estate associated with that (not in real life, but something I had dreamed about several times over the years). This ordeal was partially to me as repentance to making things hard for him years ago and he was going to get even.

They had arranged an exercise consisting of fishing line hooked into the ceiling fan and a toy soldier attached and I had to feed or unwind the line to enable the toy to not reach the fan or floor, nor to cause the fan motor to burn out. Hours on hours was spent on this while sweating profusely and not getting any relief, while my arms were numb from constant use. I was sitting in my recliner manipulating my whole body as if I was pulling in a fishing net, but with nothing in my hands. The only relief came when the girl I had stood up for years ago and some of the other women involved said that it was detrimental to my health to keep going for so long without rest. Other little games and exercises were done to keep me on the edge and not knowing what was happening, always using the good cop bad cop routine on me, just as I would get ready to stop the exercises.

When my daughter and grandson came over one day, I was constantly rolling my hands together like I was winding up cord. She kept asking me what I was doing and my grandson kept telling her to leave me alone and to leave while I tried to explain that I had been rolling up twine and felt like it was still in my hands. I also kept seeing things written all over the walls, ceilings, new furniture, windows, rugs, everywhere and in every room. Name calling about me and June and family, threats, etc.

I didn't want my family to notice so I urged them to leave after dropping meals off before their eyes caught some of the writings. They were camouflaged into the patterns of the products they were written on, but stood out vividly to me, once I could see them. I even tried my best to wash some of them off, until I thought all was ruined, but obviously there was nothing there.

They showed videos and pictures on the TV constantly to embarrass me, but they were barely visible to me and not totally recognizable, but believable to me, and I was told the identity of each individual as they appeared, because I couldn't really identify them.

Family and friend events that were all made up to wear me down as the places and events were not memorable to me. Police events that never happened, hung over my head and the cop who looked like me made up to impersonate me in old and new fake scenes. All of us doing unmentionable activities in many different locations, some with family and some with friends. There was also a house alarm constantly sounding that I begged them to turn off because I was worried about it hurting Maggie's ears and it was starting to drive me crazier (I even continued to hear it on the way to the hospital and for hours in the hospital).

My family didn't hear it when they were here, nor was it heard by hospital staff, since it was just in my head. At one point they told me I had had a sexual encounter with three of the women which I knew wasn't true and not even possible, but I was shown a video where they drugged me and had their way with me and I couldn't even remember it, and didn't believe it was me in the video, but it was supposedly video taped right there with me in my chair. They watched me in the bathroom and joked back and forth at how shy I was. Told me I couldn't flush the toilet because the septic was full and I was going to be charged with that along with other infractions I had incurred and that they would take my house from me because of everything wrong with it and my inability to fight for it.

At one point I thought my whole family was here watching all the videos in disgust and disbelief, and my sister in law got mad at me and stormed out of the house because it was messy. On the way to the hospital they told me that she had made a petition to have June's body exhumed and have an autopsy and was going to move the grave to their family plot in Wilmington. I told my son this while he was driving with his kids in the back, and he said "Dad, you have Mom's ashes right on your fireplace, none of this is real, she's not even buried." I acknowledged that fact, felt relieved by it, and within a few minutes I still believed everything else was real. Somewhere during these few days, the dream of June still being alive had been discarded.

While at hospital I was acting like a fool to get attention so that someone might recognize me and help me. Dancing and singing in bed, creating a scene with a male nurse telling him to put a catheter in because I had to pee and they wouldn't let me leave the bed. He gave me a urinal but I couldn't go so finally they did put a catheter in as I had a lengthy wait for a room, or evaluation. The voices told me they were sending two of the girls to push me through the in processing faster. I was told to look behind me, I did, and there were two of the girls from the fortune telling table dressed as candy stripers helping with the testing, one of them my old friend from our youth. I was told they were doing an MRI of my brain and checking my ears and they might find the electronics. The voices sounded worried, and I chided them for getting into this situation that would expose them. I was given a hearing test and heard the voices throughout the entire test but still passed the test and the MRI's were negative, thoughts of my head exploding relinquished. I kept hearing them for the entire time at the hospital and they directed my every response.

Multiple doctors and nurses kept asking me about it and I finally said it was fading away, but it wasn't. My Oncologist intervened and let me leave again, a few days after my fever dissipated and I began to act somewhat normal, but continued to hear the voices. They would always wake me by chanting "Bubba, Bubba, Bubba until I would acknowledge them. Then the questions would start and the prodding would continue. Your Doctor is really pretty, why don't you grab her and kiss her when she comes over. That nurse is pretty too. What is the matter with you, don't you like women anymore. They like you, go ahead and do something. That Doctor is an idiot and doesn't have a clue, they are going to find the implants in your eyes and ears and on and on and on.

My kids thought I may have taken too many opioids but I never even took what my prescription allowed and it didn't show up in my toxicology tests, nor did the doctors concur. I can describe in great detail all of these events and how it was affecting me and my relationships with everyone else, but I am only describing a small portion of them, and still remember them in great detail. I had decided that I could never let anyone know to what extent this occurred, because they would think I was seriously flawed. The hallucinations didn't continue after the girls in the hospital, however the voices never left. They did dissipate over time, but continued to pop up occasionally to let me know I'm still occupied and they are always ready to mess with and control me.

THIRD HOSPITAL ADMISSION, 8/20/16

Hallucinations and voices started taking me over again about one week before I went to the hospital. My kids were sensing something and were keeping in touch on a more timely basis because I wasn't feeling well, was acting strangely again, and the 4th anniversary of June's passing had just come and gone.

It started this time with me hearing little lawn care jingles, like commercials. They began getting more loud, directly related to my neighbor's business, and more importantly inviting me to participate in a subliminal way to improve them. After a few episodes/days, I began to realize that it was beginning again and I went over to see my neighbor and asked him to please end it before it got worse. Of course he didn't know what I was talking about and asked if I was OK. I told him I was fine, just didn't want this ordeal to begin again. He naturally called my son and Chris came over and quizzed me about the situation. I told him that I know he didn't believe it but I was alright and would get it under control. The kids began to bring me meals again and caution me to not take too much medication and to go get help if I needed it.

The voices escalated over the next few days and things started picking up where they had left off a few years earlier, only in a more dramatic way. The same characters were in play, but as the days passed, that group increased probably two to three fold. There was now an entire syndicate of the original group and some new characters, plus a lot of relatives and friends and business associates/customers that I have known throughout my life. As the days began to roll by, again without much sleep or food, but much more physical and mental involvement than before, a new plot began to unfold for me. The strange part was that most of the new characters didn't come to fruition until I had come back home from the two hospital stays of almost two weeks total. And several overall themes came to light before that transition and became clarified after coming home and starting my recuperation.

Similar events began early on including the night visits and carnival type productions. This time however they were accomplished by a separate crew who set it up in the house and the yard in the middle of one night, as I watched thinking I was not noticed. Again I was being monitored completely and everything I had improved and added to our home over the thirty plus years, was under scrutiny and inspection. I was harbored almost entirely in my sunroom as people were brought in to make inspections of everything. I was told that my house was condemned and had been sold to my neighbor without my knowing they had had it condemned for multiple reasons. As the story unraveled, I found out that my lot and adjoining properties were all being bought up or taken in similar fashion because there was an oil deposit beneath the surface. There was a competing contract for the entire area by a conglomerate that was going to build a giant medical and hospital complex to serve the entire county. This group was unaware of the oil reserve and was being muscled out by many individuals primarily in the home building/real estate acquisition business.

A few more days of deprivation and mind games and I could tell I was getting weaker and weaker. The final episode with the carnival atmosphere started when I was getting at the end of my ropes and I was told that I would be able to see and talk to June. I'm not real clear about how long this took to play out, but it wound up that she was presented to me in a hallucination and seemed to be a hallucination to me during the hallucination.

She was somewhat disguised and I was in the seat of a ride similar to a kids roller coaster and she was standing behind me with her arms around me and hugging me. She had appeared from a foggy entrance in the ceiling, I couldn't see her full face but had the vision of watching from another perspective and could tell it was her by her voice and actions. We started uphill on a journey through a cloud-like atmosphere at a walking type speed and through various curtains, lights, music, fog, and other noises I can't remember. We were expressing our feelings for each other and how great it would be to be together again and began turning up and down and round and round. As we seemingly were coming back to the start, we passed through several compartments in which were different females loosely dressed trying to seduce me and pull me away from June. I ignored them totally and asked June not to pay attention to them. Each compartment and female became more provocative and seductive, until June and I both broke down in tears.

I can remember sobbing hysterically, my "supporters" consoling me and telling the others to stop and June disappearing up into the cloudy atmosphere holding her arms out to me. The next thing I remember is laying in my bed on my left side and crying and having a hard time breathing. My neighbors voice began informing me that I had been duped into that state with drugs and deception by his boss, who were both behind and in control of me.

This was the first time I have a recollection of him saying he was working for others. He wouldn't tell me who but said I knew him. I remember struggling to move and couldn't. I was told that I was being subdued from behind and being administered some type of infusion that was going to take my life. More verbiage continued for some time as I got weaker and weaker and less lucid. A countdown was started and I started trying to escape from whatever and whoever was trying to kill me.

I finally succeeded breaking free but still had bindings and couldn't get out of bed as I heard someone running down the hall and a door slamming shut and Maggie barking loudly as I was fighting out of bed.

As I finally got up, very groggy, I was told the name of an individual that I had met years earlier who owned a building and development business was the one holding me there and taking my property. I was also told there was no way to stop that and if I really wanted to be with June, the only way was for me to cut my throat and I would be back with her forever. I remember getting excited and yelling "well I can certainly do that", and ran into the sunroom with Maggie following and barking.

I opened a cabinet door and grabbed a medium sized buck knife, sat down in my recliner and sliced from right to left with the knife, then sliced left to right. It felt like a finger cut, sort of a burning feeling, and I sat a minute and felt to see how much blood was coming out of the cuts. It didn't feel like it was enough, so I picked the knife back up and cut diagonally across the two previous cuts in an X fashion. The knife edge seemed to catch into one of the other cuts and pull at the skin which did hurt, but I finished, feeling like maybe the knife wasn't sharp enough. I saw a real sharp folding knife on my coffee table that I used to cut oranges and apples as snacks, grabbed it and drew it across my left wrist while the blood started flowing and I think I cut part of a tendon because it hurt to move my hand. I just sat in the chair for a while as I was being told that I did the right thing, but it was going to be a problem for my family and friends.

I came to the realization that I should call for help but was told no. As I continued to fight with myself, I put towels on the wounds to try and stop the bleeding and tried both phones and computer but couldn't get a connection. During the proceeding sessions with the voices, they had convinced me that they had disconnected my phones and computer and that I was at their mercy contacting anyone. I had worked and worked on all of them to no avail and was sure that they were not operational, but tried anyway, without success.

The voices told me that if I wanted help they would call the police so I told them OK and just sat back and dozed in the chair. Later they told me they cops were outside, but couldn't get in. I saw flashing lights out back and heard voices. It was the cop from before and he wasn't doing anything but waiting till it was over. I thought I heard other voices talking to him and I grabbed a flashlight from the table and pulled aside the shade a little to shine it out of the window to signal, but didn't have enough energy to get out of the chair. Frustrated I dozed off as the voices kept joking about the situation I had gotten myself in.

Next, the voices said they would come over and take me to the ER. More time went by until they admitted that they couldn't do that because it would expose them, but would call 911. Nothing…I became frustrated and mad and said I would get someone myself. I got myself out of the chair with the towels around my neck and arm and got to the family room door with my truck right outside. I'm guessing this was one to two hours after I had made the cuts which was between 10 and 12 midnight, August 20, 2016, my daughter Shannon's 43rd birthday and was aware she was celebrating her birthday at the Delaware Park Casino for the evening and would not be home until late morning.

I started getting woozy and decided to use my key fob to start the truck and initiate the horn and flashers. I did that off and on for another period of time trying to keep Maggie away from my wounds laying on the rug in front of the door. Living in the country and having scarce neighbors and little late night traffic, no help came. I told the voices that I was going to drive myself to the ER and they said I couldn't which made me more intent on doing it. I pulled myself up made it to the car barefooted I believe, dressed in the shorts and shirt I had worn for the past several days of my voice occupation. I got in and kept telling myself to stay awake, drive slow, and not attract any attention. I made it the approximately 6 miles to the ER, parked the car out front and walked past the startled security guard and nurse/receptionist stationed in the lobby area handed her my car keys, while she and a few others helped me into a treatment room, sat me down to start work along with asking me what had happened to me. I told them that I had done this to myself because I was being held and manipulated by the man, who I did name and said he was trying to kill me, and was told I would be with my wife again if I did this.

I demanded to talk to the state police because the local police were involved and was trying to tell them all about the episode. I was frantic, loud and abusive with my language and kept insisting the police find the man. The last thing I remember is getting a shot and seeing a woman I recognized starting work on my neck, another man working on my wrist and then I blacked out, all within a few minutes of walking in there.

I awoke some time later in a hospital bed and very groggy. A few nurses were wondering in and out and I was just squinting out of my eyes trying to assimilate my thoughts. I began to realize that I was strapped down and was intubated and very uncomfortable. I laid there, watching the routine of the nurses as they moved in an out of the room and as soon as one left again, I began fighting silently to get out of the bindings. I was able to break my right arm out and immediately and slowly pulled the tube out of my throat, which was very uncomfortable, and started to work on my left arm. Just then, a nurse came in and yelled for help. All of a sudden I had several people fighting to hold me down while I fought and cursed them out and demanded to talk to the police and to see my family, counselor or doctor. I also wanted to know where I was because I didn't recognize the rooms that I had become very familiar with over the last four years with my wife's and my Mother's hospitalizations, as well as my own long stays.

I was told I was at the local hospital in the intensive care unit, but I thought I was being lied to because I didn't recognize the view from the window and none of the information on the posted daily schedule board. I began thinking I was somewhere else and thought it might be the work of my voices trying to keep me confused and isolated. I had a feeling I was not being told the truth and I remember the voices scarce at that time other than chastising me for driving there.

I was assigned sitters to stay with me constantly and began talking to them and building a rapport with them. I remember three young trainees and one older gentleman that work part time. I was very comfortable with them, trying to fix up my grandson with one from the Dominican Republic and another that was the twin of a girl Chris dated in high school, both real people and conversations. That morning, I regained my senses and sought out familiar faces of the nurses to apologize from cursing at them, letting them know that was not my norm. I was able to apologize to about three and was very thankful they had not taken it personally and said they were used to that sort of thing. Two of them over the next few days got very talkative and helpful with me and wanted to really understand what was going on with me, as well as the sitters that I encountered.

I did my best to inform them of my ordeal from my diagnosis, my wife's illness and passing as well as my Mom. I also told them briefly about the voices and they wanted to know more. All along, the voices telling me not to say anything. The older gentleman was very religious and took a strong interest in me and suggested that it was the devil working against me and all I had to do was prove to him that I was religious. I told him that I had not been religious since my first few months in Vietnam, even after growing up with a grandfather that was a baptist preacher and at one point thinking I wanted to preach too.

Being desperate to stop the voices, the next day I started to try and convince the voices that I was religious. I kept repeating what the old guy told me in my head and felt like it was working for a while, even took the time to thank him as we watched countless hours of TV together, and he offered a suggestion for me to hire him to help around the house and visit with me after discharge. After about half a day the voices started making fun of me and told me that no one knew I was even in the hospital and that I couldn't fool them with my fake stories.

I had been trying to get the staff to contact my family but could not remember any phone numbers since they were all on direct dial. Also asked them to get ahold of my VA doctor and counselor or my oncologist. Time went by and I heard from no one. The voices told me that I didn't drive myself, but my neighbor took me and met my best friend from 30 years work, at the hospital which was hard to believe since I had not corresponded with her for a few days.

We usually emailed each other every week or so since my retirement seven years earlier, but that wouldn't have given her any idea I was in trouble. I knew that I had been in recent email contact with another good friend from my childhood and we were to meet for lunch that Monday (I was admitted Sunday AM). We were both Vietnam vets but had not really talked together about it for years and were finally starting to catch each other up.

Not an easy thing for either one of us as we had both kept most of our experiences to ourselves for 45 years. We had both gone through some hard and similar life changing events recently, such as having to be caregivers for our mothers, and decided we needed each other as confessors, to whatever extent necessary. He emailed me on Monday to verify our lunch date and obviously got no reply from me.

My son and daughter had been trying to raise me via phone and computer the previous few days and finally called the police to report me missing after checking the house and finding my truck gone. The police met them to fill out a missing person report and got into the house and discover the blood and knives. The police called the hospital and found out that I had driven myself there and had obviously left Maggie unattended.

My son checked the phones and computer, found nothing wrong with them and found the message from my old friend from grade school. My daughter emailed my friend to let him know what had happened and he let some other friends know. I also had a scheduled appointment with my counselor for that Monday and she called my son when I missed the appointment. She was actually in the hospital that day attending another emergency of one of her patients and couldn't leave him to see me. When she finally tried to see me, they wouldn't let her in because I was in ICU and she wasn't family. My kids came to see me that Monday or Tuesday evening loaded with questions to which I didn't really have any concrete answers other than the voices.

That led me to the hardest thing I ever had to do which was to apologize to my kids, grandkids and friends that I was sorry that I had tried to kill myself. That morning I realized that the woman I recognized in the ER was June's surgeon from the breast cancer who repaired my neck wounds and was the physician in charge of my case. June and I had a very good rapport with her and she knew of the difficulty I was having because of my illness and June's passing and quietly informed me that the VA was going to require me to admit myself into a mental facility for testing. I told her I understood and thanked her for being considerate and quiet about it.

It took two days to have the paperwork completed, and find an opening for me and I was moved during the night to the VA Mental facility in West Chester, PA, via ambulance. I was strapped in and it was a horrible bouncing ride that took almost 3 hours because the drivers got lost, as a result, the unit was short staffed early in the morning. I was slowly interviewed by three individuals the final being a Psychiatrist, in between emergency situations, deloused along with my clothes and walked by escort about a block to my ward. I was given a double room for the rest of the night and didn't sleep a wink because my roommate was deeply snoring. The voices were gaining more and more control of me as time passed and I was isolated by not knowing a soul or really where I was other than the name of the facility.

My 10 days or so at the VA hospital was like a step backwards in time for me as to the daily routines. And the feeling of complete aloneness, as I had felt entering the army. Stand in line for meals, vitals, medications, doctors visits, nurses attention, telephone (very limited to use and time, one per ward), haircuts, group sessions, etc. There were mandatory group sessions, gatherings and one TV, controlled by group decision. I had to go through a meeting with approximately 10 doctors, nurses and specialists every morning and stand up and detail why I was there and answer questions for roughly 45 minutes, followed by several individual sessions with members of that group, who would verify my stories via telephone with my son.

Most of the patients, of about 30 male and female, were there for drug addiction and were 30 years old and under. I was certainly not the oldest, but one of them. Most were there on multiple self-admissions, some wounded, most not, while I was on my first and ONLY!

I was being told what I could eat and not, when I could go somewhere and not by the voices, constantly. I was even tested in keeping my eyes open constantly without blinking while sitting in the group tv room, and not allowed to fall asleep. I could not sleep at night, because of the snoring and tried to sing favorite songs silently in my head, in order to sleep. Often the voices tried to assist my falling to sleep in a gesture of good will and my old grade school friend who had a lovely voice, but got irritated and stopped when they thought it should have worked in a certain amount of time and didn't, which prompted the desire to keep me awake.

I had some comforting conversations with a few of the other patients to the point which we shared our reasons for being there.   One young woman who was a heavy and recurring drug user, a young soldier seriously wounded in

Afghanistan and confined to a wheel chair, recuperating and too involved in opiates for pain, and an older (approximately my age) Latino, who spoke little English and reminded me of the big Native American in the old movie, "One Flew Over The Cukoo's Nest".

I developed a sincere liking for some of them because they were all alone and had no outside support group, and became very dissatisfied with myself for not using the great support group I had. I expressed this in some of the self-help groups as well as my group meetings with the professionals. I felt very cheap for doing what I did without considering the consequences to my family and friends, especially two grandsons who had lost a best friend recently to suicide. It was very hard to apologize to the two of them, which they accepted graciously and very adult like.

I was very honest in my depictions of the ordeal and claimed that I now believed that the voices represented my conscience, and likely I had been going through that most of my life, but to a lesser extent and certainly not a conscious decision, but indeed a revelation to me. I have always challenged myself when coming up against those life situations that we all do. I historically look back and opine on the decisions I have made or am making. Maybe more than most, maybe not. I do go backwards and try to make mistakes right on many occasion, but certainly not all.

I have had a static noise in my ears/head since returning from Vietnam and have always attributed it to the explosions and artillery on fire bases and base camps endured during my tour. Occasionally that static would give way to music or even something similar to a radio or tv broadcast, or simply slight voices.

Those slight voices or transmissions incorporated into the voices I began hearing during that second hospitalization and increased and amplified exponentially as time passed. The periods between and after the second and third hospitalization has not been void of the voices or the feeling of being manipulated, or at least the threat of manipulation. I was constantly reminded they were there by the calling of my name and the subtle challenge of something I was thinking or maybe an alternate way of thinking to make me think about whatever was being considered or said.

I became very used to listening to the voices while communicating with others, as it was constant. Occasionally and especially in the beginning, I would talk out loud to them until I was cautioned to stop that as I might make a mistake and answer the voices out loud. An example like eating dinner with Shannon and her family, being told what I could eat and how much, while Shannon is serving me, and me having to appear to get seconds while actually removing food. Even to the point of rehearsing questions doctors might ask me. The voices and my refutes were constant while awake. There seemed to be no escape except for sleep, and adequate sleep, came very hard. I tried putting earphones on and listening to music, meditation and even Native American chants and instruments, very loud! They were still there, but subdued to an extent.

The voices woke me or were there upon awaking. I stood my ground with them often and refused to comply with their "orders", part of my natural and stubborn streak. There were penalties that were usually administered in reductions of awards achieved along the way, like demerits. Towards the end, my intended total destruction had transformed into a brand new estate with all expense trips for a plane load of friends and family to Hawaii, a

Dolphin vs Patriot football game in Miami, new cars, an airplane, a job with a prominent political figure (stemming from a mutual friend who was his right hand man and teammate from Delaware football and a plane ride with him from Las Vegas to Philadelphia for June and I, and finally a meeting with Chris and the politician's people for an Annapolis Appointment).

New cars for me and grandsons, and on and on with a running dollar total. All of these and pieces of them were continually added and taken away as I performed favorably or not so much! The subject matter in each of these areas I was tested, can be born from my actual life experiences. I bring a few up to prove that point and I'm sure I could do it for each situation if pressed. Of course the further up I progressed, the more my mind accepted it to be more of a mind game from one end of the spectrum to the other. Maybe that is why it stopped. Where else could it go?

Back to the end of the stay in the hospital for the third time. Finally after about 10 days I was released and my son drove up to take me home the next day. My daughter and her sons had arranged to have my rugs shampooed because of the situation I left Maggie in. She also went through the house and made it presentable to me, so I walked into a welcoming environment and an excited Maggie. My main goal was to make everything right for everyone, and my 24/7 roommate Maggie got most of the attention. I had lost some weight because I wasn't allowed to eat and Maggie had lost some as well due to the change in her routine. They certainly fed her and walked her, but not in the regiment that I had built with her and because of her lack of cooperation. We worked hard to get that back in line, that is why I wouldn't play along with the voices about not touching and talking to her, and both ended up considerably lighter and hopefully more healthy.

HOME RECUPERATION

As part of the VA follow up of suicide attempts, I had to meet with a member of the assigned team every week for about three months. The team consisted of my Psychiatrist , counselor, or another assigned counselor. That process went without a problem and I am currently awaiting an appointment with my new Psychiatrist soon, as mine left the VA for greener pastures. I continue to meet with my counselor monthly and via telephone in between if needed and have a very solid relationship with her, a much needed relationship on my part. I have several friends from 35 to 60 years ago that pretty much know everything about me, but my counselor probably knows and understands me better, especially the last five years.

My neighbor's group was stealing the properties well below cost by faking documentation to each landowner and had accomplices within the government. Their end game to force out the hospital group by offering more money and causing less area politics. Their intention to develop the extraction of oil on a low scale, unobtrusive plan while converting the entire acreage into executive mansion/properties for those involved and families (approximately 2-3 square miles of mostly non developed woodlands within the boundaries of four roads). If I were to choose to fight this change I would be eliminated with an unfortunate accident or bought out as were the other homeowners and landowners.

Many details that I had discovered over the years since 1983 when we bought the property were brought back into my mind. The fact that all properties on my side of the road were divided into precise two acre rectangles with two access areas between my property and my southern neighbor and another toward the north end of the road. These access areas to provide future access to the wooded areas behind our properties and the nucleus of the rough center area between these two roads. I assumed the situation was similar on all four of the roads which enclosed the original property.

I had discovered the access area when I had researched the property surveys back in 1983 and identified the original landowner and current owner of the predominate land to be one V. P. The area between my neighbor and our lot was 50' X 440' approximately and was a parallel lane between both lots accessing the center property. Then other access from my road is one lot over to the other side. I had further researched the surveys and contacted the owner by phone in 1983 and requested his permission to maintain the property that bordered my southeastern property line as there was an existing drainage ditch roughly on the extreme edge of the line. My neighbor had a partial fence near the edge of his line and I asked to take care of the ground on my side. The owner agreed because he said he didn't expect to ever sell that land and I noted the conversation on my copy of my survey.

I assume this was the basis of the information stored in my brain which allowed this elaborate scheme to be hatched. Many, many other relationships and incidents and personalities from my childhood, through college, the Army, and most of my working career came into this mix in my head to blend in with the story. It seems that any questions I might have brought up to myself and choices I must have been troubled about along the way, were brought up through the creation of these ordeals. Exaggerated and amplified over and over to be as confusing but possibly believable to this confused state I was in.

As the constant back and forth exchanges continued, more and more individuals and separate schemes began to develop, but mostly after I began my recuperation at home following my release from the hospital, as were the examples described earlier.

The circumstances started changing from getting me out of the way to wanting to utilize me because of the connections and relationships I had with many other individuals. I can only assume that was because I had made it through the attempted suicide which changed the outcome in my mind. I started to be challenged to change in ways they wanted to work together for the entity, even being told that I could win a lot of money by becoming the fastest "text typer" and could win a rigged state lottery that was also being controlled by people in my past that had multiple connections.

I was then schooled in the game of liars' poker which I had a brief explanation while in the army. I was offered to let Chris become my proxy and he would enter a big regional game with a fixed hand that I was actually holding with cash of all denominations in my house. This was also part of the crooked lottery system of which a friend of Chris' from HS and her mother were involved. The girl used to be a cheerleader and actually became a Miss Delaware and June and I knew her parents through the HS Boosters clubs. This little ploy played out over days intertwined with other schemes and tests ongoing, involved at least twenty five people who were all intertwined and constantly talking individually and in groups.

We even involved spirits of relatives and close friends for consultative input. We never got to the end of most of the games or whatever they were, but they were always part of the loss or gain for me on the tally sheet.

I began training around the clock on my typing skills using anything with a keyboard, even air typing and eventually won the contest against an old friend and computer/software writer. Convenient right? (I took typing in 9th and 10th grades and by the time I finished was the second fastest/accurate typist in the school. Only one senior girl could beat me. I started on manual typewriters and finished on electric units. I continued typing through college, typing my own term papers and others for a slight charge. During my OJT after NCO school at Fort Benning, I was assigned to a unit comprised mostly of returning Vietnam soldiers and did a lot of typing and also typed a good bit in jobs at Chrysler and when consulting.)

A gigantic web of people and associations began playing out around the clock and was very hard to keep straight. I was tested all day and night, put through yoga like trances, sometimes dressed in shirt and tie and sometimes nude.

My son was attempting to keep me on medications at that point after my return home from the hospital and witnessed quite a few of those examples and I believe took pictures of same. I was tasked with many foolish schemes to wear me down, like throwing myself against walls, falling like I was dead from a walk, over and over again until I did it convincingly. I won't describe them all at this time or in detail because they are both embarrassing and too revealing, but I can do so in vivid detail.

Such as searches for hidden treasures, secrets, pictures, etc. throughout the entire house including attic and crawl space, outside buildings and shrubbery. I was told to throw all of my house phones away (7) and did so as well as destroying my cell, which I threw as hard as I could against the wall. I later found all but two of the phones and some months later while planting an small garden, I found the other two overgrown with grass. I even ordered parts and cleaned them to revive them.

I was told to break some decorative Buddha statues I had and did that to two but stopped after I threw the broken ones out in the front yard with other items as instructed by the voices, which Chris found a day or so later. I was told I had so many seconds to run to the pole barn without clothes, open it and find some hidden money. I tried, but ruined my toes because I was barefoot, on gravel and it was fall and hundreds of acorns and monkey balls were on the ground. I also have very tender feet from the neuropathy caused by my years of chemo. I started out with flip flops, but can't wear them because I have no control grip with my toes because of the neuropathy. That is all they would allow me to wear.

I wasn't allowed to talk to Maggie or to comfort her with touch after coming home from the hospital, but that only lasted a very short time because I couldn't and wouldn't do it. I had to sleep on the floor nude next to her for days. I had to conceal my medications and spit them out after Chris dispensed them to me. I had to dress in suit and tie and wait outside for a helicopter to pick me up. Of course it never came. I was told that there was an "eye in the sky" that could monitor everything I did outside in addition to the coverage they had me under inside, even showed how it works on the computer. I had to wear a tie around the house on some days, occasionally without a shirt, when Chris came by so I had to give him an explanation. There is no question I was being led to making my kids believe I was crazy, because I was so afraid they would put me away.

My first day home I called both Shannon and Chris and asked to meet with them. I begged them to not allow me to be put I into that situation again because I would not be able to take it. They were totally caught off guard. Chris had arranged while working with my VA counselor to be put on a Hospice plan when I returned home.

Something was confusing about that to me because Hospice to me , by connotation, meant that it was an end of life phase that I had just undergone with June 4 years earlier. I had the first meeting and felt very uncomfortable with the discussion. I checked in with my counselor and found there was some sort of misunderstanding among someone. When the second meeting came with Hospice, I was asked to sign papers. I told them my concerns and they said it wasn't the same as with June, but I couldn't get a comfortable feeling and declined to sign or to be a part. They called into their office, had a hushed conversation and packed up and left. Later that week, I received via UPS the same medical/pharmacy package I had received for June. I still have both and they are identical. I didn't have to use June's kit as it is an emergency backup if no response is answered by hospice medical staff.

I still don't understand that whole situation. I just knew and explained to my counselor that I was not in that bad of shape to need to entertain the program. Never heard another word about it.

*While I am thinking it right now I will mention that these happenings were going 24/7, at least in my mind, for all of these events and that is the main thing that wore me down, along with feeling ill and having a mild fever during the beginning phases. So there is much, much more detail than I am including in these notes that I recall verbatim in many cases, as mentioned earlier. I realize all of this was concocted in my subconscious mind and much was derived from my past and my dreamlike creativity.

More importantly, it truly seemed real to me, even when my son, primarily, but others also, had convinced me it was all in my mind. An extreme recollection that my head might explode during an MRI if there was really something implanted in me. It didn't scare me, but I did think about it and knew it would prove something positive to understand the reality of what was happening to me, that it was just in my mind. This is probably one reason I convinced myself that I was just reasoning with my conscious and trying to make myself believe I was doing the good/right thing.

Listening to that good angel instead of the bad one on the other shoulder. I also wonder how many people suffer similar, if not as desperate issues or worse, while trying to do the right thing with their life during trying times or while deliberating about choices to make. I am pretty well convinced that my subconscious mind has generated all of these incidences or whatever they are from my memory or thoughts or dreams, fears, wishes etc., over the years. Instances in my life or my being that I had to make a decision to do or not do, just like everyone else has to contend with throughout their lives. Whether they are real or not, these experiences truly felt real at the time.

I probably have always questioned myself on decisions of the heart and mind but these examples went overboard. I still weigh most things I am deliberating quite thoroughly now, at least it is much more recognizable to me since these past experiences. Have I always been like this, but not recognized the distinct back and forth arguments within myself? I really don't know! It has now been just over a year and half since I was last admitted to the hospital. The voices continued until a few months ago, now I am back to the constant static in my ears/mind and the constant arguing with myself via talking to myself physically (when alone) or through thoughts. Trying to do what is right for myself as well as others.

I have accomplished more in the last year and half than I did in the almost six years June has been gone, at least physically. June and I worked the flower gardens together from spring through fall and I took care of the grass and the household projects with her design, furniture moving, tear out and painting help.

I stopped all flower garden work, her bathroom renovation, and future projects the day she came home under Hospice. I neither physically or mentally felt competent nor capable to continue. I did what I could to keep the house and yard acceptable and her bathroom approximately 20% completed, which she never saw.

I had planned to surprise her with her dream bathroom. A fairy theme, with walk in tub, elevated toilet, walk in shower steam bath and marble topped double vanity. I had the master bedroom bath to use for myself and had completed the heated tile floor, glass block wall, curtains and toilet installed when I stopped. She saw the tile completed and picked out the curtains from choices I let her choose colors from. She saw the vanity and top and tub in the garage, but nothing in place, because I hadn't finished the plumbing and separate water installations yet.

I had everything designed in my head and in drawings I had made, but anyone that knows me knows that those things change until the day it is finished or even changed later and in progress. We also had new tile picked out to remodel the kitchen and sitting in the garage and I had just finished remodeling the brick fireplace with marble tiles when she went into the hospital the last time.

When she came from the hospital the first thing she asked me was if I had finished the bathroom, didn't say "my". I told her no, and Shannon asked if she wanted to see it and she answered yes. She was so tired and on her last legs in the hospital bed, and there was no way other than pictures, which I wasn't in favor of. She never saw it with her living eyes, but I know she has seen it and visited it often.

It was almost four years when my counselor convinced me to finish the bathroom and I agreed with her. It took me many weeks to slowly finish everything as I wasn't mentally into it nor physically very capable, but I finally did finish it and am very proud that it is definitely one of a kind. There will never be anything close. Everything she wanted including many fairies, butterflies, birds, etc. Big mirrors, a TV behind a mirror to watch from the walk in tub or red leather chair and makeup table. Lighted glass block wall behind tub, with colored rainbow beads and triple pull out hamper beneath. Slightly obscured toilet with small curio above it and cleaning closet next to assist service to hidden TV. Six foot sliding medicine cabinet on side wall with matching drapes pulled back. Triple window with shades with pull back drapes. Double wood vanity with custom hanging mirrors. One a round copper, colored crystal flower to match copper crystal panels covering skylight, door panels. Butterfly mirror over other sink extending from glass block wall. Both mirrors with ceramic fairy paintings on the tub side and six others on walls and hampers. Lighted glass block quarter round transition from vanity to tub, and lighted glass block wall ceiling cornice to meet glass block wall and side mirror to vanity. End wall is a four foot standing glass quarter round and redwood interior shower/steam bath, with hidden dedicated water heater and towel storage shelving closing it off. Hanging crystal fixtures over sinks, crystal four unit floor lamp over tub and chair with hanging fixture matching copper over makeup table. And separate recessed lighting. Two standing heated towel racks and final decorations.

One sub note relating to the voices. Following the return home after the last hospital stay. One of the exercises I had to go through because the house was being sold was that I had to disassemble everything in the bathroom in order to sell the parts for money. Even had live auctions being conducted by the group as the disassembly was occurring and I was only given a certain timeframe to get it done, designating piles for purchasers. This just months after I had finished everything.

Chris happened over shortly afterward and wanted to know what happened and I was told to tell him I had a leak. Had only used the tub a few times because I was ordered to use it because of my neuropathy. I had all of the plumbing and access areas torn apart, including some light fixtures. I put it all back together a few days later and made some more changes to the room.

I had all of June's remaining jewelry separated and split into piles for the same reason. She had willed her most favorite pieces to the girls and I had given some to her sister shortly after her passing, but I loved giving her jewelry and there is still dozens of pieces left, which I pull out often and have some on display in the bathroom. That's the only work I had done to the house since 7/29/2012, when June came home for good, and that was only because I agreed with my counselor.

Speaking about all of the jewelry I have given her over the years for every occasion, I have to laugh about her birthday gift one of the years we were totally flooded at work after the passing of a hurricane. Most of us at work had been putting more than 12 hours a day, for about two weeks and still had another week or two just to get fully operational again.

I was dead tired, getting older and more forgetful, but luckily remembered that it was that special day, and stopped at the last convenience store on the way home and bought her two pints of her very expensive, favorite ice creams and a single rose. She told me that that was her favorite birthday present I had given her later in our lives, because I remembered it on the spur of the moment, under those conditions, and it meant more to her than anything else I could have given her. I tried it again years later, only without the problem of a flood, and didn't get the same results, but did get a laugh and had a back up gift for her to add to the collection.

As I worked myself through the next six months home from the hospital and dealing with the traumatic dealings within my head, I began trying to set new goals for myself at the urging of family, friends, and counselor. I wanted to try and open myself up a little and considered selling and moving into a smaller home. The voices had told me they would be with me at least another year or more. All I could do is try to work through it all, but dreaded them being with me, and was begging them and looking everywhere for relief.

I began reading heavily again as I found that allowed me to escape a little. Not that they went away, but at least I could loose myself a little while mentally hearing sporadically placed comments or read alongs. Later on I began watching movies on TV and trying to engross myself in them until 2-3 AM, along with the reading. I believe that over this long period, it helped me rid the voices from my head. I now keep that up, sleep in 3-4 hour or shorter batches and feel ok with it. It allowed me to get out in the yard last year and accomplish many things I had been neglecting. Gardens, finishing deck and stairs, power washing decks and house, cleaning and reorganizing garage and pole barn and getting cars organized and clean, working on lawn mower and garden equipment.

As summer weather was getting too rough for me I moved up my next project of remodeling the kitchen up a few months. I started by ripping everything out including water damaged subfloor. Ordered new cabinets, used 6 year old tile that June and I purchased, redid ceiling with wood planks, electric, plumbing, paint, laundry room and pantry and added tile backsplash over brick chimney and countertops. New ceiling fan and recessed and pendant fixtures and of course subbed out granite sink and countertops.

It took me three months because I cant work for long at a time or fast and I'm a whole lot weaker than I used to be, but I did finish in time to have the family for Christmas. Of course I put a few signature projects in there, like a lighted glass block corner, serving bar, and lighted crown molding. It's a small kitchen, so I have to embellish
and add my signature design features.

I've slowed down again during the winter months with my annual bout with flu like symptoms and the malaise I surrender to around the holidays and will again around the anniversary of June's passing in August. I'm trying to force myself back into the outside mode again since April is almost gone, but the weather hasn't worked with me. Yard work and cleaning away winters effects are calling me, and it has been so wet, I've been cutting close to the driveway only for Maggie, because the yard overall is just too wet. I've only gotten the leaves up, cut a bunch of downed branches, tinkered with my lawn equipment, but I'm planning a lot for the
future.

GLOSSARY/BIBLIOGRAPHY

Vietnam War Statistics

War Statistics
Protest and Kent State
A Letter to the Wall

VIETNAM WAR STATISTICS

IN UNIFORM AND IN COUNTRY...

- Vietnam Vets: 9.7% of their generation.
- 9,087,000 military personnel served on active duty during the Vietnam Era (Aug. 5, 1964 - May 7, 1975).
- 8,744,000 GIs were on active duty during the war (Aug 5, 1964 - March 28, 1973).
- 3,403,100 (Including 514,300 offshore) personnel served in the Southeast Asia Theater (Vietnam, Laos, Cambodia, flight crews based in Thailand, and sailors in adjacent South China Sea waters).
- 2,594,000 personnel served within the borders of South Vietnam (Jan. 1, 1965 - March 28, 1973)
- Another 50,000 men served in Vietnam between 1960 and 1964.
- Of the 2.6 million, between 1 - 1.6 million (40 - 60%) either fought in combat, provided close support or were at least fairly regularly exposed to enemy attack.
- 7,484 women (6,250 or 83.5% were nurses) served in Vietnam.
- Peak troop strength in Vietnam: 543,482 (April 30, 1968)

CASUALTIES...

- Hostile deaths: 47,378
- Non-hostile deaths: 10,800
- Total: 58,202 (Includes men formerly classified as MIA and Mayaguez casualties). Men who have subsequently died of wounds account for the changing total.
- 8 nurses died -- 1 was KIA.
- Married men killed: 17,539
- 61% of the men killed were 21 or younger.
- Highest state death rate: West Virginia - 84.1% (national average 58.9% for every 100,000 males in 1970).
- Wounded: 303,704 -- 153,329 hospitalized + 150,375 injured requiring no hospital care.
- Severely disabled: 75,000 -- 23,214 - 100% disabled; 5,283 lost limbs; 1,081 sustained multiple amputations.
- Amputation or crippling wounds to the lower extremities were 300% higher than in WWII and 70% higher than Korea. Multiple amputations occurred at the rate of 18.4% compared to 5.7% in WWII.
- Missing in Action: 2,338
- POWs: 766 (114 died in captivity)

DRAFTEES VS. VOLUNTEERS...

- 25% (648,500) of total forces in country were draftees. (66% of U.S. armed forces members were drafted during WWII.
- Draftees accounted for 30.4% (17,725) of combat deaths in Vietnam.
- Reservists killed: 5,977
- National Guard: 6,140 served; 101 died.
- Total draftees (1965 - 73): 1,728,344.

Vietnam War Statistics (Page 2)

- Actually served in Vietnam: 38%
- Marine Corps Draft: 42,633.
- Last man drafted: June 30, 1973.

RACE AND ETHNIC BACKGROUND...

- 88.4% of the men who actually served in Vietnam were Caucasian; 10.6% (275,000) were black; 1% belonged to other races.
- 86.3% of the men who died in Vietnam were Caucasian (includes Hispanics); 12.5% (7,241) were black; 1.2% belonged to other races.
- 170,000 Hispanics served in Vietnam; 3,070 (5.2% of total) died there.
- 70% of enlisted men killed were of North-west European descent.
- 86.8% of the men who were killed as a result of hostile action were Caucasian; 12.1% (5,711) were black; 1.1% belonged to other races.
- 14.6% (1,530) of non-combat deaths were among blacks.
- 34% of blacks who enlisted volunteered for the combat arms.
- Overall, blacks suffered 12.5% of the deaths in Vietnam at a time when the percentage of blacks of military age was 13.5% of the total population.
- Religion of Dead: Protestant -- 64.4%; Catholic -- 28.9%; other/none -- 6.7%

SOCIO-ECONOMIC STATUS...

- 76% of the men sent to Vietnam were from lower middle/working class backgrounds.
- Three-fourths had family incomes above the poverty level; 50% were from middle income backgrounds.
- Some 23% of Vietnam vets had fathers with professional, managerial or technical occupations.
- 79% of the men who served in Vietnam had a high school education or better when they entered the military service. (63% of Korean War vets and only 45% of WWII vets had completed high school upon separation.)
- Deaths by region per 100,000 of pupulation: South -- 31%, West -- 29.9%; Midwest -- 28.4%; Northeast -- 23.5%.

WINNING & LOSING...

- 82% of veterans who saw heavy combat strongly believe the war was lost because of lack of political will.
- Nearly 75% of the public agrees it was a failure of political will, not of arms.

HONORABLE SERVICE...

- 97% of Vietnam-era veterans were honorably discharged.
- 91% of actual Vietnam War veterans and 90% of those who saw heavy combat are proud to have served their country.
- 66% of Vietnam vets say they would serve again if called upon.
- 87% of the public now holds Vietnam veterans in high esteem!!!!!

http://history-world.org/Vietnam...war...Statistics.htm

Glossary of Military Terms (page 1 of D only)

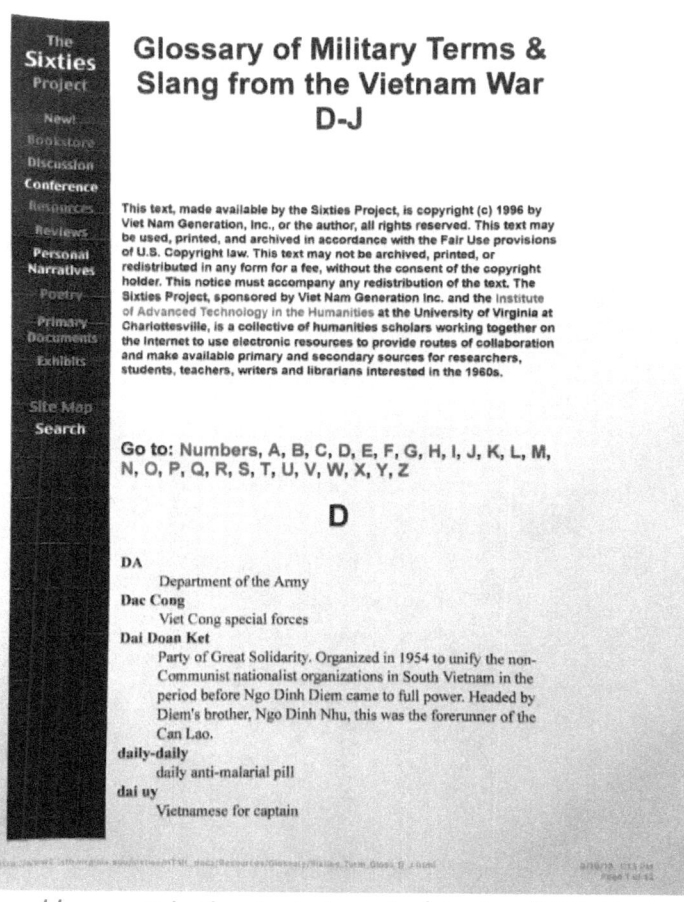

http://www2.lath.virginia.edu/sixties/HTML_
docs/Resources/Glossary/Sixties...Term...Gloss

Agent Orange-Related Illnesses

Agent Orange-Related Illnesses

We believe that contact with Agent Orange, a toxic chemical used to clear trees and plants during the Vietnam War, likely causes several illnesses. Find out if you can get disability compensation or benefits if you had contact with Agent Orange while serving in the military and now have 1 or more of the illnesses listed below.

Cancers believed to be caused by contact with Agent Orange

- **Chronic B-cell Leukemia**: A type of cancer that affects your white blood cells (cells in your body's immune system that help to fight off illnesses and infections)
- **Hodgkin's Disease**: A type of cancer that causes your lymph nodes, liver, and spleen to get bigger and your red blood cells to decrease (called anemia)
- **Multiple Myeloma**: A type of cancer that affects your plasma cells (white blood cells made in your bone marrow that help to fight infection)
- **Non-Hodgkin's Lymphoma**: A group of cancers that affect the lymph glands and other lymphatic tissue (a part of your immune system that helps to fight infection and illness)
- **Prostate Cancer**: Cancer of the prostate (the gland in men that

https://www.vets.gov/disability-benefits/conditions/exposure-to-hazardous-materials/agent-orange/diseases/

Agent Orange-Related Illnesses (cont'd)

helps to make semen)

- **Respiratory Cancers (including lung cancer):** Cancers of the organs involved in breathing (including the lungs, larynx, trachea, and bronchus)
- **Soft Tissue Sarcomas (other than osteosarcoma, chondrosarcoma, Kaposi's sarcoma, or mesothelioma):** Different types of cancers in body tissues such as muscle, fat, blood and lymph vessels, and connective tissues

Other illnesses believed to be caused by contact with Agent Orange

- **AL Amyloidosis:** A rare illness that happens when an abnormal protein (called amyloid) builds up in your body's tissues, nerves, or organs (like your heart, kidneys, or liver) and causes damage over time
- **Chloracne (or other types of acneform disease like it):** A skin condition that happens soon after contact with chemicals and looks like acne often seen in teenagers. Under our rating regulations, it must be at least 10% disabling within 1 year of contact with herbicides.
- **Diabetes Mellitus Type 2:** An illness that happens when your body is unable to properly use insulin (a hormone that turns blood glucose, or sugar, into energy), leading to high blood sugar levels
- **Ischemic Heart Disease:** A type of heart disease that happens when your heart doesn't get enough blood (and the oxygen the blood carries). It often causes chest pain or discomfort.
- **Parkinson's Disease:** An illness of the nervous system (the network of nerves and fibers that send messages between your brain and spinal cord and other areas of your body) that affects your muscles and movement—and gets worse over time
- **Peripheral Neuropathy, Early Onset:** An illness of the nervous system that causes numbness, tingling, and weakness. Under our

Page 2 of 3 (Agent Orange-Related Illnesses)

Agent Orange-Related Illnesses(cont'd)

rating regulations, it must be at least 10% disabling within 1 year of contact with herbicides.

- **Porphyria Cutanea Tarda**: A rare illness that can make your liver stop working the way it should and can cause your skin to thin and blister when you're out in the sun. Under VA's rating regulations, it must be at least 10% disabling within 1 year of contact with herbicides.

If you have an illness you think is caused by contact with Agent Orange—and you don't see it listed here—you can still apply for benefits. You'll need to show that you have a disability and include a doctor's report or a hospital report stating that your illness is believed to be caused by contact with Agent Orange.

Apply for benefits.

Page 3 of 3 (Agent Orange-Related Illnesses)

Fact VS Fiction…..The Vietnam Veteran

FACT VS FICTION……THE VIETNAM VETERAN

The stereotypes are wrong. Let's look at the facts, starting with who actually served in Vietnam.

The image of those who fought in Vietnam is one of poorly educated, reluctant draftees -- predominantly poor whites and minorities. But in reality, only one-third of Vietnam-era veterans entered the military through the draft, far lower than the 66 percent drafted in World War II.

It was the best-educated and most egalitarian military force in America's history -- and with the advent of the all-volunteer military, is likely to remain so. In WWII, only 45 percent of the troops had a high school diploma. During the Vietnam War, almost 80 percent of those who enlisted had high school diplomas, and the percentage was higher for draftees -- even though, at the time, only 65 percent of military-age males had a high school diploma.

Throughout the Vietnam era, the median education level of the enlisted man was about 13 years. Proportionately, three times as many college graduates served in Vietnam than in WWII.

Another common assumption: The war in Vietnam was fought by youngsters wet behind the ears, who died as teenagers barely old enough to shave. In fact, more 52-year-olds (22) died in Vietnam than 17-year-olds (12). An analysis of data from the Department of Defense shows the average age of men killed in Vietnam was 22.8 years, or almost 23 years old.

Though the notion persists that those who died in Vietnam were mostly members of a minority group, it's not true. About 5 percent of KIAs were Hispanic and 12.5 percent were black -- making both minorities slightly under-represented in their proportion of draft-age males in the national population.

A common negative image of the soldier in Vietnam is that he smoked pot and injected heroin to dull the horrors of combat. However, except for the last couple of years of the war, drug usage among GIs in Vietnam was lower than for U.S. troops stationed elsewhere. When drug rates started to rise in 1971 and 1972, almost 90 percent of the men who served in Vietnam had already come and gone. A study after the war by the VA showed drug usage of veterans and non-veterans to be about the same. And marijuana -- not heroin -- was the drug used in 75 percent of the cases. Of those addicted, 88 percent kicked the habit within three years of returning.

Posterboy of Anti-War Movement:

The anti-war movement paraded Vietnam servicemen who had deserted their units as "proof" that it was an immoral war. But of the 5,000 men who deserted for various causes

https://www.vvof.org/factsvnv.htm

Facts VS Fiction.....VV (cont'd)

during the Vietnam War period, only 5 percent did so while attached to units in Vietnam.

Only 24 deserters attributed their action to the desire to "avoid hazardous duty." Some 97 percent of Vietnam veterans received honorable discharges, exactly the same rate for the military in the 10 years prior to the war.

After the war ended, reports began to circulate of veterans so depraved from their war experiences that they turned to crime, with estimates of the number of incarcerated Vietnam veterans as high as one-quarter of the prison population. But most of these accounts were based on self-reporting by criminals. In every major study of Vietnam veterans where military records were verified, an insignificant number of prisoners were found to be actual Vietnam veterans.

A corollary to the prison myth is the belief that substantial numbers of Vietnam veterans are unemployed. A study by the Labor Department in 1994 showed an unemployment rate of 3 percent for Vietnam veterans -- lower than that of Vietnam-era veterans who served outside the Vietnam theater (5 percent), and for all male veterans (4.9 percent).

The same is true for the nonsense that Vietnam vets have high rates of suicide, often heard as the "fact" that more veterans had died by their own hand than in combat. But that's a myth, too. A 1988 study by the Centers for Disease Control found Vietnam veterans had suicide rates well within the 1.7 percent norm of the general population.

Societal Success:

In fact, Vietnam veterans are as successful or more successful than men their own age who did not go to war. Disproportionate numbers of Vietnam veterans serve in Congress, for instance. Vice President Al Gore is a Vietnam veteran, as is enormously popular Colin Powell.

They run Fortune 500 corporations (Frederick Smith of Federal Express), write screenplays (Bill Broyles formerly of Newsweek) and report the evening news (ABC correspondent Jack Smith).

Actor Dennis Franz, who plays a detective on TV's NYPD Blue, is a Vietnam vet, as are large numbers of real law enforcement agents, prosecutors and attorneys. No facet of American life has been untouched by the positive contributions of Vietnam veterans.

While stereotypes may persist in Hollywood and the media, America's finest increasingly run the country.

Vietnam Warriors:

Facts VS Fiction…..VV (cont'd)

A Statistical Profile In Uniform and In Country Vietnam Vets: 9.7% of their generation.
9,087,000 military personnel served on active duty during the Vietnam era (Aug. 5, 1964-May 7, 1975)
8,744,000 GIs were on active duty during the war (Aug. 5, 1964-March 28, 1973).
3,403,100 (including 514,300 offshore) personnel served in the Southeast Asia Theater (Vietnam, Laos, Cambodia, flight crews based in Thailand, and sailors in adjacent South China Sea waters).
2,594,000 personnel served within the borders of South Vietnam (Jan. 1, 1965- March 28, 1973).
Another 50,000 men served in Vietnam between 1960 and 1964.
Of the 2.6 million, between 1-1.6 million (40-60%) either fought in combat, provided close support or were at least fairly regularly exposed to enemy attack.
7,484 women (6,250 or 83.5% were nurses) served in Vietnam.
Peak troop strength in Vietnam: 543,482 (April 30, 1969).

Casualties

Hostile deaths: 47,378
Non-hostile deaths: 10,800
Total: 58,202 (includes men formerly classified as MIA and Mayaguez casualties). Men who have subsequently died of wounds account for the changing total.

8 nurses died -- 1 was KIA.

Married men killed: 17,539

61% of the men killed were 21 or younger

Highest state death rate: West Virginia- 84.1 (national average 58.9 for every 100,000 males in 1970).

Wounded: 303,704 -- 153,329 hospitalized + 150,375 injured requiring no hospital care.

Severely disabled: 75,000 -- 23,214 100% disabled; 5,283 lost limbs; 1,081 sustained multiple amputations.

Amputation or crippling wounds to the lower extremities were 300% higher than in WWII and 70% higher than in Korea. Multiple amputations occurred at the rate of 18.4% compared to 5.7% in WWII.

Missing in Action: 2,338.

Page 3 of 5

Veteran)Facts VS Fiction.....VV (cont'd)

POWs: 766 (114 died in captivity).

Draftees vs. Volunteers:

25% (648,500) of total forces in country were draftees. (66% of U.S. armed forces members were drafted during WWII.)

Draftees accounted for 30.4% (17,725) of combat deaths in Vietnam.

Reservists killed: 5,977.

National Guard: 6,140 served; 101 died.

Total draftees (1965-73): 1,728,344.

Actually served in Vietnam: 38%

Marine Corps draft: 42,633.

Last man drafted: June 30, 1973.

Race and Ethnic Background

88.4% of the men who actually served in Vietnam were Caucasian; 10.6% (275,000) were black; 1% belonged to other races.

86.3% of the men who died in Vietnam were Caucasian (includes Hispanics);

12.5% (7,241) were black; 1.2% belonged to other races.

170,000 Hispanics served in Vietnam; 3,070 (5.2% of total) died there.

70% of enlisted men killed were of Northwest European descent.

86.8% of the men who were killed as a result of hostile action were Caucasian; 12.1% (5,711) were black; 1.1% belonged to other races.

14.6% (1,530) of non-combat deaths were among blacks.

34% of blacks who enlisted volunteered for the combat arms.

Page 4 of 5

Facts VS Fiction....VV (cont'd)

Overall, blacks suffered 12.5% of the deaths in Vietnam at a time when the percentage of blacks of military age was 13.5% of the total population.

Religion of Dead:

Protestant -- 64.4%; Catholic -- 28.9%; other/none --6.7%.

Socio-Economic Status

76% of the men sent to Vietnam were from lower middle/working class backgrounds.

Three-fourths had family incomes above the poverty level; 50% were from middle income backgrounds.

Some 23% of Vietnam vets had fathers with professional, managerial or technical occupations

79% of the men who served in Vietnam had a high school education or better when they entered the military service.
(63% of Korean War vets and only 45% of WWII vets had completed high school upon separation.)

Deaths by region per 100,000 of population: South-31; West-29.9; Midwest-28.4; Northeast-23.5.

Winning & Losing

82% of veterans who saw heavy combat strongly believe the war was lost because of lack of political will.

Nearly 75% of the public agrees it was a failure of political will, not of arms.

Honorable Service

97% of Vietnam-era veterans were honorably discharged.

91% of actual Vietnam War veterans and 90% of those who saw heavy combat are proud to have served their country.

66% of Vietnam vets say they would serve again if called upon.

87% of the public now holds Vietnam veterans in high esteem.

Page 5 of 5
https://www.vvog.org/factsvnv.htm

Operation Lam Son 719 Operation S. Laos Campaign (8 February to 25 March 1971 Page 1 only of 27 available)

Operation Lam Son 719 or 9th Route - Southern Laos Campaign (Vietnamese: *Chiến dịch Lam Sơn 719 or Chiến dịch đường 9 – Nam Lào*) was a limited-objective offensive campaign conducted in the southeastern portion of the Kingdom of Laos. The campaign was carried out by the armed forces of the Republic of Vietnam (South Vietnam) between 8 February and 25 March 1971, during the Vietnam War. The United States provided logistical, aerial, and artillery support to the operation, but its ground forces were prohibited by law from entering Laotian territory. The objective of the campaign was the disruption of a possible future offensive by the People's Army of Vietnam (PAVN), whose logistical system within Laos was known as the Ho Chi Minh Trail (the Truong Son Road to North Vietnam).

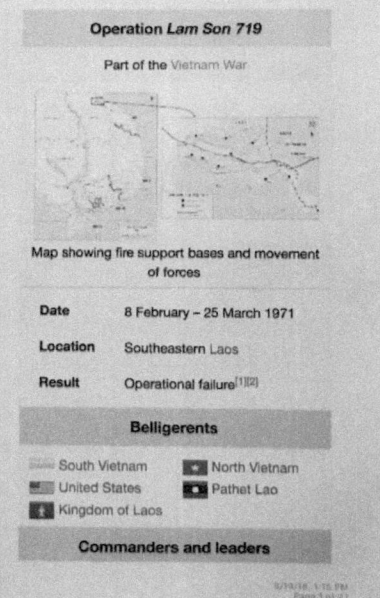

Operation *Lam Son 719*
Part of the Vietnam War

Map showing fire support bases and movement of forces

Date	8 February – 25 March 1971
Location	Southeastern Laos
Result	Operational failure[1][2]

Belligerents

South Vietnam — North Vietnam
United States — Pathet Lao
Kingdom of Laos

Commanders and leaders

https://en.m.wikipedia.org/wiki.Lam...Son...719

My Lai Massacre (Page 1 only of 48 available)

"My Lai" redirects here. For the hamlet, see Sơn Mỹ. For the documentary, see My Lai (film).

The **Mỹ Lai Massacre** (/ˌmiːˈlaɪ/; Vietnamese: *Thảm sát Mỹ Lai*, [tʰâːm ʂǎːt mǐˀ lāːj] (listen)) was the Vietnam War mass murder of unarmed Vietnamese civilians by U.S. troops in South Vietnam on 16 March 1968. Between 347 and 504 unarmed people were massacred by the U.S. Army soldiers from Company C, 1st Battalion, 20th Infantry Regiment, 11th Brigade, 23rd (Americal) Infantry Division. Victims included men, women, children, and infants. Some of the women were gang-raped and their bodies mutilated.[1][2] Twenty-six soldiers were charged with criminal offenses, but only Lieutenant William Calley Jr., a platoon leader in C Company, was convicted. Found guilty of killing 22 villagers, he was originally given a life sentence, but served only three and a half years under house arrest.

The massacre, which was later called "the most shocking episode of the Vietnam War",[3] took place in two hamlets of Sơn Mỹ village in Quảng Ngãi Province.[4] These hamlets were marked on the U.S. Army topographic maps as Mỹ Lai and Mỹ Khê.[5]

The U.S. Army slang name for the hamlets and sub-hamlets in that area was *Pinkville*,[6] and the carnage was initially referred to as the *Pinkville Massacre*.[7][8] Later, when the U.S. Army started its investigation, the media changed it to the *Massacre at Songmy*.[9] Currently, the event is referred to as the *My Lai Massacre* in the United States and called the *Sơn Mỹ Massacre* in Vietnam.[10]

Mỹ Lai Massacre
Thảm sát Mỹ Lai

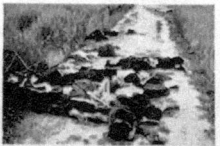

Photo taken by United States Army photographer Ronald L. Haeberle on the 16th of March, 1968 in the aftermath of the Mỹ Lai massacre showing mostly women and children dead on a road.

https://en.m.wikopedia.org/wiki/My.Lai. Massacre

Definition: accelerationism

In political and social theory, **accelerationism** is the idea that either the prevailing system of capitalism, or certain technosocial processes that have historically characterised it, should be expanded, repurposed, or accelerated in order to generate radical social change. Some contemporary accelerationist philosophy takes as its starting point the Deleuzo-Guattarian theory of deterritorialisation, aiming to identify, deepen, and radicalise the forces of deterritorialisation with a view to overcoming the countervailing tendencies that suppress the possibility of far-reaching social transformation.[1] Accelerationism may also refer more broadly, and usually pejoratively, to support for the deepening of capitalism in the belief that this will hasten its self-destructive tendencies and ultimately lead to its collapse.[2][3]

Accelerationist theory has been divided into mutually contradictory left-wing and right-wing variants. "Left-accelerationism" attempts to press "the process of technological evolution" beyond the constrictive horizon of capitalism, for example by repurposing modern technology for socially beneficial and emancipatory ends; "right-accelerationism" supports the indefinite intensification of capitalism itself, possibly in order to bring about a technological singularity.[4][5][6]

Background

A number of philosophers have expressed apparently accelerationist attitudes, including Karl Marx in his 1848 speech "On the Question of Free Trade":

> But, in general, the protective system of our day is conservative, while the free trade system is destructive. It breaks up old nationalities and pushes the antagonism of the proletariat and the bourgeoisie to the extreme point. In a word, the free trade system hastens the social revolution. It is in this revolutionary sense alone, gentlemen, that I vote in favor of free trade.[7]

In a similar vein, Friedrich Nietzsche argued that "the leveling process of European man is the great process which should not be checked: one should even accelerate it...",[8] a statement often simplified, following Deleuze and Guattari, to a command to "accelerate the process".[9]

http://en.m.wikipedia.org/wiki/Accelerationism

Outpatient Oncology Drug Series: Doxorubicin Is the Infamous Red Devil
(Page 1 only of 9 available)

Outpatient Oncology Drug Series: Doxorubicin Is the Infamous Red Devil

April 10, 2015 by Jill Weberding (/author/jill-weberding) BSN, MPH, RN, OCN®

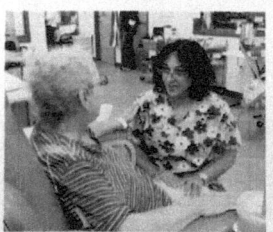

Editor's note: This article was first published on April 10, 2015, and updated on May 29, 2018.

https:// life.ons.org/news-and-views/outpatient-oncology-drug-series-doxorubicin-is-the-Infamous-red-devil

www.ingramcontent.com/pod-product-compliance
Lightning Source LLC
Chambersburg PA
CBHW020638220526
45464CB00001B/202